Small Animal Ophthalmology:
A Problem-oriented Approach

SANDERS /HANSEN

To our families

Small Animal Ophthalmology: A Problem-oriented Approach

Second Edition

Robert L. Peiffer Jr
DVM, PhD, DipACVO
Professor, Departments of Ophthalmology and Pathology,
School of Medicine, University of North Carolina, Chapel Hill, USA

Simon M. Petersen-Jones
D Vet Med, DVOphthal, DipECVO, MRCVS
RCVS Specialist in Veterinary Ophthalmology
Department of Clinical Veterinary Medicine,
University of Cambridge, UK

W.B. SAUNDERS COMPANY LTD
London Philadelphia Toronto Sydney Tokyo

W. B. Saunders Company Ltd	24–28 Oval Road London NW1 7DX, UK
	The Curtis Center Independence Square West Philadelphia, PA 19106–3399, USA
	Harcourt Brace & Company 55 Horner Avenue Toronto, Ontario M8Z 4X6, Canada
	Harcourt Brace & Company, Australia 30–52 Smidmore Street Marrickville, NSW 2204, Australia
	Harcourt Brace, Japan Ichibancho Central Building, 22–1 Ichibancho Chiyoda-ku, Tokyo, 102, Japan

© 1997. W. B. Saunders Company Ltd

A catalogue record for this book is available from the British Library

ISBN 0–7020–2017 6

First edition published 1989
First edition translated into French, German and Japanese.

Phototypeset by J&L Composition Ltd, Filey, North Yorkshire
Printed and bound in Great Britain by Jarrold Book Printing Ltd, Norfolk

Contents

Contributors

P G C Bedford BVetMed PhD DVOphthal DipECVO MRCVS
Professor and Head of Department, Department of Small Animal
Medicine & Surgery, The Royal Veterinary College (University of
London), Hatfield, Hertfordshire, UK

Ellen Bjerkås DVM PhD DipECVO
Associate Professor, Department of Small Animal Clinical Sciences,
Norwegian College of Veterinary Medicine, Oslo, Norway

Cynthia S Cook DVM PhD DipACVO
Veterinary Vision – Animal Eye Specialists, San Mateo, California,
USA

Björn Ekesten MScVM PhD
Research Fellow, Department of Medicine and Surgery, Swedish
University of Agricultural Sciences, Faculty of Veterinary Medicine,
Uppsala, Sweden

B H Grahn DVM DipABVP(CA) DipACVO
Associate Professor, Ophthalmology, Department of Veterinary
Internal Medicine, Western College of Veterinary Medicine,
University of Saskatchewan, Saskatoon, Canada

R Gareth Jones BVSc CertVOphthal MRCVS
The Park Veterinary Group, Whetstone, Leicester, UK

Kristina Narfström DVM PhD DipECVO
Professor, Department of Medicine & Surgery, Swedish University of
Agricultural Sciences, Faculty of Veterinary Medicine, Uppsala,
Sweden

Robert L Peiffer Jr DVM PhD DipACVO
Professor, Departments of Ophthalmology & Pathology, School of
Medicine, University of North Carolina at Chapel Hill, Chapter Hill,
USA

Simon M Petersen-Jones DVetMed DVOphthal DipECVO MRCVS
RCVS Specialist in Veterinary Ophthalmology, Department of Clinical
Veterinary Medicine, University of Cambridge, Cambridge, UK

Claudio Peruccio DVM DipECVO
Professor of Companion Animal Diseases, Department of Animal
Pathology, Faculty of Veterinary Medicine, University of Torino,
Italy

Stefano Pizzirani DVM DipECVS
Medico Veterinario, Clinica Verinaria 'Europa', Florence, Italy

Peter W Renwick MA VetMB DVOphthal MRCVS
Willows Referral Service, Shirley, Solihull, West Midlands, UK

Jeffrey S Smith BSVc FACVSc DipACVO
Animal Eye Clinic, Cremorne, New South Wales, Australia

Richard I E Smith BSVc FACVSc
Department of Companion Animal Medicine & Surgery, University
of Queensland, Queensland, Australia

Robin G Stanley BSVc (Hons) FACVSc-Ophthalmology
Animal Eye Care, East Malvern, Australia

J Wolfer DVM DipACVO
Veterinary Referral Clinic of Mississuga, Mississauga, Ontario,
Canada

Preface to First Edition

Ophthalmology has blossomed and matured as a recognized, valued specialty of veterinary medicine and surgery; ophthalmic exposure is generally emphasized in the professional curriculum; the competency and sophistication of the general practitioner is continually improving; and several excellent contemporary comprehensive textbooks are available on the subject.

Then why this text? We have recognized a need by the general practitioner for an informative source that he or she can turn to as a guide to the management of a particular problem. Appropriate management implies two inseparable principles – accurate diagnosis and adequate therapy. We have attempted to address each with equal emphasis. We perceive a need by the student for a text that condenses a large amount of information into a 'friendly' manual that emphasizes problem solving rather than memorization and that provides more usable information than lecture notes without the depth of a reference text. We hope this manual meets these needs.

Why these authors? The profession and the specialty are evolving and changing. Although I am somewhat reluctant to classify myself as 'mature' as a clinical ophthalmologist, I cannot help but be impressed by the energy, enthusiasm, and ideas of a younger generation of amazingly well-trained ophthalmologists. All of the contributors fit this mold, and I hope that they and their colleagues who follow will continue to probingly question the established as well as addressing unsolved problems. Experience is almost always tainted by dogmatism, which in turn can cloud truth; I have encouraged Drs. Cook, Leon, Cottrell, and Petersen-Jones to express their ideas and philosophies without unwarranted respect for sacred cows. The product is exciting.

We have attempted not to reproduce a comprehensive text but to produce a clinical manual; references are not included. As conditions may present with more than one presenting sign, there is some repetition; conditions are discussed in detail under their most obvious or significant sign. We have discussed in detail only those surgical procedures that are likely to be routinely performed by the practitioner, and details of these procedures are described with their pictorial presentation rather than in the text. Emphasis is placed on techniques that have proven to be most valuable and effective for the authors, and readers should recognize that there may indeed be quite acceptable alternative approaches to clinical problems. We do hope that this handbook will prove a ready and valuable reference to the general practitioner presented with a challenging ophthalmic case and when reviewed in its entirety will provide a practical overall approach to small animal ophthalmology.

Robert L. Peiffer, Jr.
Chapel Hill, N.C.

Preface to Second Edition

Exciting things have been happening in veterinary ophthalmology between editions of this work. The text was created to provide the small animal practitioner with a concise but comprehensive guide to the management of his or her patients that was both practical and economical, with emphasis on conceptualization and problem solving rather than a cookbook approach to clinical cases. Response to the First Edition, which was translated into three languages (French, German, and Japanese), has influenced us to update the text in an attempt to produce a work of equal but more contemporary usefulness.

The authorship of this Second Edition is truly international, reflecting the growing importance of ophthalmology as a specialism in many countries across the world. A blending of the wisdom of experienced and renowned specialists with the enthusiasm of more youthful ophthalmologists will, we hope, provide the reader with broad and stimulating perspectives. We have attempted to retain the original informal style and format, as well as the original objectives. As with the first text, the individual chapters are the personal statements of the authors – readers should recognize that there may indeed be quite acceptable alternative approaches to clinical problems, the text reflecting those philosophies and techniques that have proven to be most valuable and effective for the authors.

ROBERT L. PEIFFER, JR.
Chapel Hill, N.C., USA

SIMON M. PETERSEN-JONES
Cambridge, UK

Acknowledgements

Ophthalmology is a fascinating and multifaceted speciality. We are honoured to be given the opportunity to attempt to convey some of our enthusiasm for the subject to a wider audience. The dedication, expertise and interest of all the authors needs recognition from us as editors and we are sure that they will join with us to acknowledge the help and encouragement we have all received from our mentors and colleagues, and the support provided to us by our families.

Of course this project would not have got under way without the backing of the publishers and would never have been completed without the skills and professionalism of the publisher's employees who have turned our writings, photographs and drawings into final text.

1

Clinical Basic Science

Cynthia S Cook and Robert L Peiffer, Jr.

OCULAR EMBRYOLOGY

The ocular primordia appear during the first weeks of gestation as bilateral evaginations of the neural ectoderm of the forebrain. These optic sulci gradually enlarge and approach the surface ectoderm as optic vesicles connected to the forebrain by the optic stalks. Thickening of the overlying surface ectoderm to form the lens placode (Figure 1.1 a and b) occurs as a result of inductive influences by the optic vesicle. Invagination of the lens placode occurs concurrently with that of the optic vesicle to form a hollow lens vesicle within a bilayered optic cup (Figure 1.1 c and d), the inner layer of which will form the stratified layers of the neural retina and the inner epithelial layer of the iris and ciliary body; the outer layer becomes the cuboidal monolayered retinal pigment epithelium, the outer epithelial layer of the iris and ciliary body, and the pupillary sphincter and dilator muscles (the only muscles in the body of neural ectodermal origin). The stalk attaching the lens vesicle to the surface ectoderm gradually thins through a combination of cell death and active migration of cells out of the stalk (Figure 1.1 e and f).

Invagination to form the optic cup occurs eccentrically, with formation of a slit-like opening called the optic (choroid) fissure located inferiorly (Figure 1.1 f). The vascular supply to the embryonic eye, the hyaloid artery (primary vitreous), enters the optic cup through this opening and branches extensively around the lens to form the tunica vasculosa lentis. Embryonic remnants of this vascular structure may persist as a persistent hyperplastic primary vitreous (PHPV) and/or persistent tunica vasculosa lentis (PTVL). Failure of the optic fissure to close normally may result in congenital defects anteriorly (iridial coloboma) or posteriorly (chorioretinal or optic nerve coloboma). Microphthalmos may occur as a result of deficiencies in the early formation of the optic sulcus or vesicle or from incomplete closure of the optic fissure with failure to establish early intraocular pressure.

The posterior lens epithelial cells elongate, forming primary lens fibers that obliterate the space within the lens vesicle. Secondary lens fibers are formed by elongation of cells at the equator (lens bow); these fibers pass circumferentially around the embryonal lens

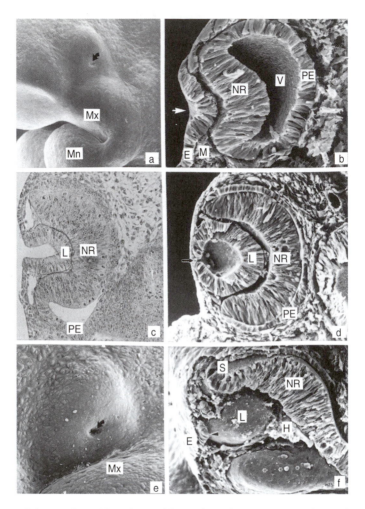

Figure 1.1   (a) Day 10 embryo (29 somite pairs). on external examination
the invaginating lens placode can be seen (arrow). Note its position relative
to the maxillary (Mx) and mandibular (Mn) prominences of the first visceral
arch (magnification = 53×). (b) Embryo of the same age as (a). Frontal
fracture through the lens placode (arrow) illustrates the associated thickening
of the surface ectoderm (E). Mesenchyme (M) of neural crest origin is
present adjacent to the lens placode. The distal portion of the optic vesicle
concurrently thickens, as the precursor of the neural retina (NR), while the
proximal optic vesicle becomes a shorter, cuboidal layer which is the anlage
of the retinal pigmented epithelium (PE). The cavity of the optic vesicle (V)
becomes progressively smaller (magnification = 184×). (c) The epithelium
of the lens placode continues to invaginate (L). There is an abrupt transition
between the thicker epithelium of the placode and the adjacent surface

nucleus. Note that the sutures are associated only with the fetal and adult lens fibers.

Thickening of the future neural retina occurs with segregation into inner and outer neuroblastic layers. Cellular proliferation takes place in the outer neuroblastic layer with migration to the inner layer. The ganglion cells are the first to achieve final differentiation, extending axons that form the nerve fiber layer and join as the optic nerve. The horizontal, amacrine, and Müller cells also differentiate in the inner neuroblastic layer. The bipolar cells and photoreceptors develop in the outer neuroblastic layer and form the inner and outer nuclear layers in the adult. Retinal dysplasia may result from disorganized development of the neural retina with formation of folds and rosettes. The retinal pigment epithelium is the determining factor for the differentiation of the layers on each side, namely the retina and the choroid and sclera.

Following detachment of the lens vesicle from the surface ectoderm, development of the anterior chamber structures progresses. A specialized population of the neural ectoderm called the *neural crest cells* migrates under the surface ectoderm to form the corneal endothelium which secretes its basement membrane, Descemet's membrane. Additional neural crest cells form the corneal stroma between the surface epithelium and endothelium. The anterior iris stroma also develops from neural crest cells migrating onto the anterior surface of the optic cup. Neural crest cells also form the outer two coats of the posterior globe, the choroid (including the tapetum) and sclera.

---

ectoderm, which is not unlike the transition between the future neural retina (NR) and the future pigmented epithelium (PE) (periodic acid Schiff's; magnification = 221×). (d) As the lens vesicle enlarges during day 11, the external opening, or lens pore (arrow), becomes progressively smaller. The lens epithelial cells at the posterior pole of the lens elongate to form the primary lens fibers (L). NR = anlage of the neural retina; PE = the anlage of the pigmented epithelium (now a very short cuboidal layer) (magnification = 150×). (e) External view of the lens pore (arrow) and its relationship to the maxillary prominence (Mx) – 32 somite pairs (magnification = 130×). (f) Frontal fracture reveals the optic fissure (*) where the two sides of the invaginating optic cup meet. This forms an opening in the cup allowing access to the hyaloid artery (H) which ramifies around the invaginating lens vesicle (L). The former cavity of the optic vesicle is obliterated except in the marginal sinus (S), at the transition between the neural retina (NR) and the pigmented epithelium. E = surface ectoderm (magnification = 154×).

(Reprinted with permission from *J. Vet. Comp. Ophthalmol.* 1995; **5**: 109–123).

OCULAR ANATOMY, PHYSIOLOGY, AND BIOCHEMISTRY

Orbit

The orbit in the cat and dog is formed by contributions of the frontal, palatine, lacrimal, maxillary, zygomatic, and presphenoid bones. The bony orbit is incomplete superiotemporally, where it is bridged by the dense orbital ligament, spanning between the frontal process of the zygomatic bone and the zygomatic process of the frontal bone. The lacrimal gland lies superiorly, under this orbital ligament. The orbital contents are covered by a connective tissue layer of periorbita, which is continuous at the limbus with Tenon's capsule. Seven extraocular muscles innervated by the third, fourth, and sixth cranial nerves control movement of the globe. There is a variable amount of fat between the periorbita and the bony wall and surrounding the extraocular muscles. The zygomatic salivary gland is located inferiotemporally, deep to the zygomatic arch, and may be a site of infection or mucocele formation.

The wall of the bony orbital wall is thinner medially and may allow extension of infectious or neoplastic processes originating in the nasal cavity or periorbital sinuses. Infectious processes involving the roots of the molar teeth may also extend to involve the orbit.

Space-occupying orbital lesions include both inflammatory and neoplastic etiologies. Due to the incomplete nature of the bony orbit, both inferiorly and superiotemporally, a space-occupying process may become quite advanced before exophthalmos and/or deviation of the globe is noted. Diagnosis and management of such conditions are discussed in subsequent chapters.

Eyelids

The eyelids form the initial barrier to mechanical damage to the eye. They also serve to distribute the tear film and, through the meibomian glands, provide an oily secretion to slow tear evaporation. The eyelids consist of:

1. An outer layer of thin, pliable skin
2. A small amount of loose connective tissue containing modified sweat glands and the circumferential fibers of the orbicularis oculi muscle (innervated by branches of the facial nerve)
3. The more rigid fibrous connective tissue of the tarsal plate
4. The radial fibers of the levator palpebrae superioris (innervated by the oculomotor nerve) and Müller's (sympathetic innervation via branches of the trigeminal nerve) muscles
5. The palpebral conjunctiva containing goblet cells.

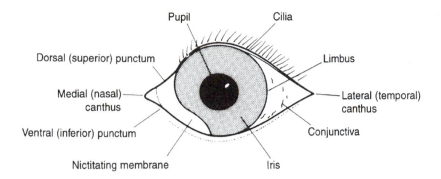

Figure 1.2 External appearance of the canine eye (with the exception of the pupillary shape, the feline is identical) depicting the adnexal structures.

Cilia are found on the margin of the upper lid; posterior to these follicles are the openings of the sebaceous (meibomian) glands (Figures 1.2 and 1.3). Dysplasia or metaplasia of these glands results in formation of aberrant hair follicles (distichia), which may contact the cornea and result in epiphora and, rarely, keratitis.

Surgical manipulations of the eyelids require delicate handling to minimize swelling and careful apposition of surgical or traumatic wound margins. Particular attention should be paid to maintenance of a smooth eyelid margin. Closure of full-thickness defects should utilize a two-layer pattern; the tarsal plate has the greatest strength and should be included in the subcutaneous layer.

Lacrimal System

The precorneal tear film consists of three distinct layers: (1) a mucus layer located closest to the cornea and produced by the conjunctival goblet cells, (2) a thick aqueous layer, and (3) an outer oily layer produced by the meibomian glands of the eyelids. The aqueous portion of the tear film is the combined product of the orbital lacrimal land and a gland located at the base of the third eyelid. The major lacrimal gland is located in the superiotemporal area of the orbit beneath the orbital ligament and supraorbital process of the frontal bone; its secretions appear through numerous small ducts in the superior fornix. The tears are distributed over the surface of the cornea through the action of the eyelids and exit through the nasolacrimal puncta. These two openings are located nasally, superior and inferior to the medial canthus, just inside the eyelid margin (Figure 1.2). The puncta open into two canaliculi joining to form the nasolacrimal duct, which passes through a bony canal in the maxilla to open ventrolaterally in the nasal cavity.

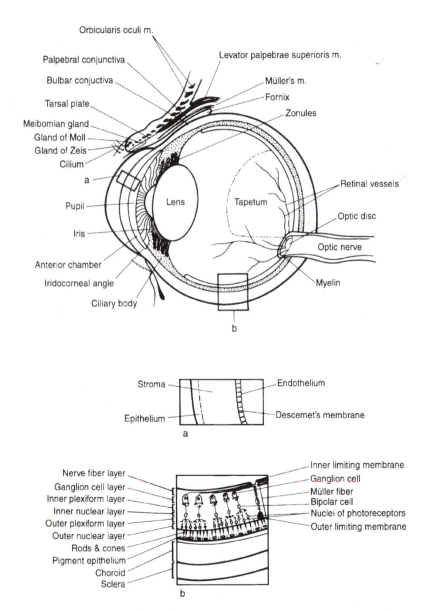

Figure 1.3   Schematic anatomy of the canine and feline eye.

Conjunctiva and Third Eyelid

The *conjunctiva* is a mucous membrane that covers the globe between the fornix and the cornea, the third eyelid, and the inner surface of the eyelids (Figure 1.3). Over the surface of the globe, the conjunctiva blends with Tenon's capsule, which attaches firmly to the limbus. The conjunctiva is a highly vascular, delicate tissue containing many mucus-secreting goblet cells. The vascularity and mobility of the conjunctiva can be used to the surgeon's advantage to act as a graft for corneal defects. The conjunctiva is also a site of localization of lymphocytes and provides a reservoir of immunocompetent cells for the globe, in particular the avascular cornea.

The *third eyelid* is a mobile, semi-rigid structure located inferionasal to the globe (Figure 1.2). It is covered on both palpebral and bulbar surfaces by conjunctiva. The third eyelid owes its rigidity to a T-shaped piece of hyaline cartilage located within its substantia propria. At the base of the cartilage is a seromucoid lacrimal gland that produces approximately one third of the precorneal tear film. Poorly defined connective tissue attaches the gland and base of the cartilage to the sclera and periorbita inferiorly. Inadequacy of these attachments with prolapse of the gland occurs not uncommonly, particularly in the American Cocker Spaniel and English Bulldog breeds. Removal of the gland in such cases is contraindicated as it may predispose to future development of keratoconjunctivitis sicca; the gland should be repositioned and sutured in place as described in Chapter 4 (p. 64).

Cornea

The *cornea* is the transparent, avascular anterior portion of the outer fibrous coat of the eye (Figure 1.2). The cornea consists of surface epithelium, collagenous stroma, and Descemet's membrane, which is the basement membrane produced by the inner endothelial monolayer. As the cornea is avascular, its oxygen and nutritional needs are met by diffusion externally from the precorneal tear film and internally from the aqueous humor; the peripheral cornea is also oxygenated by the limbal capillary plexus. Corneal transparency is a product of several factors unique to corneal physiology. Relative dehydration of the cornea is maintained by an active Na^+-K^+ ATPase-associated pump mechanism within the endoth elial monola yer. The regular arrangement of the collagen fibrils in the corneal stroma minimizes scattered light and thus enhances transparency. The normal absence of pigment and blood vessels in the stroma is also a requirement for optical transparency.

The cornea has remarkable healing capabilities. Simple epithelial defects are covered by a combination of sliding of adjacent cells and mitosis to restore normal cell number. Wounds that extend into the stroma heal first by re-epithelialization, with a longer period of time required to fill the stromal defect. Corneal scarring is a result of the irregular pattern created by replacement collagen fibrils. Vascularization is expected to accompany any corneal injury or inflammatory condition that persists longer than seven to ten days and contributes to the opaque granulation tissue that initially fills a deep corneal wound. Descemet's membrane is elastic and tends to resist tearing during an injury. Wounds extending to Descemet's membrane (descemetocele) and full-thickness lacerations are indications for immediate surgical management. Some regenerative properties are attributed to the canine endothelium, little to the feline.

Iris and Ciliary Body

The iris and ciliary body comprise the anterior portion of the middle, vascular coat of the eye, called the *uvea* (Figure 1.3). The iris creates a pupillary opening of variable diameter to adjust the quantity of light that is able to pass through the lens to reach the photosensitive retina. This variable aperture is maintained by the sympathetically supplied radial dilator muscle and the parasympathetically supplied circumferential sphincter muscle. Both muscles are located on the posterior side of the iris, deep into the pigmented epithelial layer. The iris anterior to these muscles consists of a loose, vascular connective tissue that is variably pigmented. Full-thickness corneal wounds often seal with iris tissue, which must be replaced into the anterior chamber (if viable) or excised. Surgical manipulations of the iris are frequently accompanied by hemorrhage that may complicate post-operative healing. Electrocautery may be used to control hemorrhage.

The *ciliary body* is the posterior continuation of the iris and consists of an anterior portion called the *pars plicata* (with the ciliary processes) and a posterior portion called the *pars plana*. The ciliary body is covered throughout by a bilayered epithelium of which only the deeper layer is pigmented. Aqueous humor is produced by the ciliary epithelium through a combination of passive ultrafiltration and active secretion involving carbonic anhydrase. The passive production of aqueous humor is influenced by mean arterial blood pressure. Inflammation of the anterior uvea will result in reduced active aqueous secretion and thus lowered intraocular pressure. The stroma of the ciliary body contains the smooth fibers of the parasympathetically innervated ciliary muscle, which is important in accommodation of the lens for near vision.

Aqueous humor circulates from the ciliary processes in the posterior chamber of the eye, through the pupil, to exit via the trabecular meshwork of the iridocorneal angle. During this process, metabolites are exchanged with the avascular lens and cornea. Morphologic or physiologic barriers to aqueous circulation and outflow are responsible for elevations in intraocular pressure (glaucoma).

Lens

The *lens* is a transparent, biconvex structure anchored equatorially to the ciliary body by collagenous zonule fibers (Figure 1.3). Contraction of the ciliary muscle alters the degree of curvature of the lens, thereby changing its optical power. The lens is surrounded by an outer capsule; deep to the anterior portion of the capsule is a monolayer of cuboidal epithelium. These epithelial cells are metabolically very active and undergo mitosis throughout life. As the cells multiply they move to the equator of the lens where they elongate and gradually lose their nucleus and other organelles to form the spindle-shaped lens fibers. These fibers are added in a circumferential arrangement so that older fibers are within the deeper portion of the lens. The fiber ends meet anteriorly at the upright Y suture and posteriorly at the inverted Y suture.

The anterior epithelial cells utilize glucose, which diffuses into the lens from the circulating aqueous humor and is broken down anaerobically to lactic acid. Saturation of the normal pathways for glucose metabolism occurs in diabetes mellitus and results in accumulation of sorbitol within the lens. Sorbitol attracts water, which results in a clinically observable cataract that usually progresses rapidly.

Retina

The *retina* is a complex photosensory structure consisting of ten layers: (1) pigment epithelium, (2) photoreceptors (rod and cone outer segments), (3) external limiting membrane (Müller cell processes), (4) outer nuclear layer (photoreceptor nuclei), (5) outer plexiform layer, (6) inner nuclear layer (nuclei of Müller, amacrine, horizontal, and bipolar cells), (7) inner plexiform layer, (8) ganglion cell layer, (9) nerve fiber layer (axons of ganglion cells), and (10) inner limiting membrane (Müller cell processes) (Figure 1.3). The principal neuronal connections of the retina involve the photoreceptors, which synapse with the bipolar cells which then synapse with the ganglion cells in the inner plexiform layer. The axons of the ganglion cells form the nerve fiber layer and join to make up the optic nerve at the posterior pole. The amacrine and horizontal cells form internal connections between bipolar cells and may thus exert a regulatory influence. Müller cells are a non-neuronal constituent that forms a supporting matrix and the barriers of the inner and outer limiting membranes.

Inherited retinal degenerative processes initially involve the photoreceptors, either rods, cones, or both. With time the condition usually progresses to involve the other retinal layers, and diffuse thinning and blindness results.

Tapetum

The *tapetum* is a modification of the choroid located deep to the pigment epithelium and chloro capillaris. It is composed of a highly organized arrangement of crystals containing zinc and riboflavin, which results in a reflective appearance. The color of the tapetum ranges from green to blue to yellow and varies with the species, breed, and age. Thinning of the overlying retina (as occurs in retinal degeneration) results in a hyper-reflective appearance of the tapetum.

Optic Nerve and Central Visual Pathways

The optic nerve consists of combined axons of the ganglion cells and is surrounded by all three meningeal layers of the central nervous system. The optic disk is the origin of the optic nerve within the globe; its irregular triangular appearance in the dog is a result of the variable quantity of myelin surrounding the optic nerve (Figure 1.3). The optic nerve exits the orbit at the optic foramen. The right and left optic nerves meet at the optic chiasm, located rostral to the pituitary gland. In cats and dogs, the majority (65–75%) of nerve fibers cross in the chiasm to travel as the optic tracts to the contralateral geniculate nucleus. This decussation is responsible for coordinated bilateral vision as well as the occurrence of a consensual pupillary light response (Figure 1.4).

The majority of axons in the optic tracts terminate in the lateral geniculate nucleus, synapsing on neurons whose axons form the optic radiations and terminate in the occipital cortex. This pathway is responsible for conscious visual perception.

The remaining optic tract axons bypass the lateral geniculate nucleus and terminate in the rostral colliculus of the pretectal area. Parasympathetic axons originating here synapse in the oculomotor nucleus of the midbrain, origin of the oculomotor nerves, whose axons synapse in the ciliary ganglion prior to entering the globe as the short ciliary nerves to the pupillary sphincter muscles. This pathway is responsible for the direct and consensual pupillary light responses.

Sympathetic control of the pupillary dilator muscle originates in the hypothalamus the axons from which synapse with preganglionic neurons in the first four segments of the thoracic spinal cord. These axons join the sympathetic trunk terminating in the cranial cervical ganglion. Postganglionic fibers travel to the eye after crossing the roof of the middle ear cavity and are distributed to the ciliary muscle, pupillary dilator, third eyelid, and the Müller's muscle of the upper

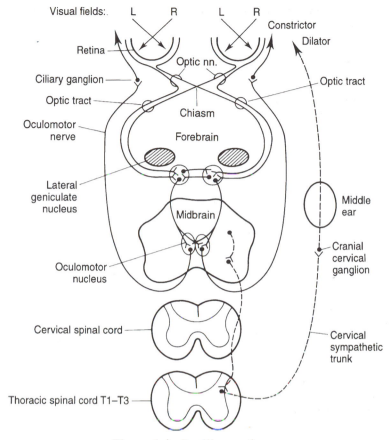

Figure 1.4 Pupillary pathways.

lid. Compromise of sympathetic innervation to the globe results in the classic signs of Horner's syndrome: ptosis (drooping of the upper lid), miosis (pupillary constriction), and protrusion of the third eyelid.

OCULAR PATHOLOGY

The systematic examination of surgical and necropsy obtained ocular tissue is essential for optimal patient management, the career-long educational process, and enhancing understanding of ocular disease in animals. Maximal benefit is obtained from optimally fixed tissues; in almost all cases, immersion fixation in 10% formalin is adequate. Fixation should be expedient as the retina especially undergoes rapid autolysis; trimming of periocular tissues enhances penetration of fixatives, and injection of 0.5 ml of the fixative into the vitreous cavity with a 27 guage needle at the equator will minimize neuro-sensory retinal separation artifact. Otherwise, submit globes intact so that the pathologist can appreciate the intertissue relationships. Use adequate volumes of fixative (at least 100 ml for dog and cat eyes), and allow 72 hr for fixation to occur.

Ocular Response to Disease

A detailed discussion of ocular pathology would fill a text of its own; principles and concepts of importance to clinicians are discussed with particular disease processes throughout the following chapters. Two related features warrant note: (1) the propensity of the ocular tissues (especially the epithelia of lens, uvea, and retina, but also the corneal endothelium and uveal vasculature) to undergo reactive changes of hypertrophy, hyperplasia, and metaplasia (in the case of feline ocular sarcomas, perhaps neoplasia as well); and (2) because of the dependence of the ocular tissues on tissue transparency and intertissue relationships for normal function, the devastating effect that these changes can have on vision. A focus of hepatitis may resolve with scarring and minimal if any functional significance, while a comparable process in the eye may lead to blindness.

Fibroplasia in the cornea, for example, will result in scarring and opacification. In the anterior chamber, peripheral anterior and posterior synechia and membranes are associated with secondary glaucoma. Iris neovascularization, also known as rubeosis irides or pre-iridal fibrovascular membrane, is a common cause of intraocular hemorrhage and secondary angle closure glaucoma. Hypertrophy, hyperplasia, and metaplasia of lens epithelium are an integral part of cataractogenesis, and the bane of the cataract surgeon who has to deal with postoperative capsular fibrosis. Vitreous detachment, fibrosis, and neovascularization lead to cyclitic membranes and their dire consequences of retinal detachment and phthisis bulbis. The clinical ophthalmologist wages a relentless pharmacologic battle against these processes with antiinflammatories and antimetabolites, and new approaches will undoubtedly play an important role in the future management of ocular disease.

2

Diagnostics

Claudio Peruccio, Stefano Pizzirani and Robert L. Peiffer, Jr

INTRODUCTION

The ophthalmic examination combined with history and signalment provide the foundation for obtaining an accurate differential diagnosis. Ophthalmic diagnosis is achieved by a combination of basic knowledge, mastering of simple instrumentation, and critical observation. The former includes an understanding of anatomy, physiology, and disease mechanisms. Instrumentation facilitates critical observation; quite basic equipment and simple techniques, including a magnifying loupe, bright focal illumination, Schirmer tear test, diagnostic dyes, cytology, direct ophthalmoscopy, and Schiøtz tonometry should be readily available in any practice, and in experienced hands will be adequate to manage the great majority of ophthalmic cases. More expensive and sophisticated instrumentation, including the biomicroscope, indirect ophthalmoscope, applanation tonometry, electrophysiology, gonioscopy, ultrasound and other imaging techniques, fluorescein angiography, and retinoscopy represent the next level of diagnostics and are available to specialists or to those with a particular interest in the field. A systematic approach to examination should be followed individually for each case based upon history and signs. Technical competency in diagnostics is achieved simply by practice and making an ophthalmic examination a part of every routine physical examination will hone skills for the occasion upon which they are more urgently required.

INSTRUMENTS AND BASIC DIAGNOSTIC TECHNIQUES

Magnifying loupe

A binocular magnifying loupe of 2× to 4× magnification, and a focal length of 15–25 cm, is useful not only for diagnostics, but surgery as well; it allows freedom of both hands for manipulation and a loupe-mounted diffuse illuminator facilitates observation as well.

Focal illumination

A transilluminator provides the optimal light for external eye examination and to test the pupillary light reflexes (PLRs). For the latter, it is important to use a narrow beam of bright light with a constant source of energy (such as a rechargeable handle) directed toward the posterior pole. One of the most common causes of abnormal PLRs is weak batteries!

Schirmer Tear Test (STT)

This test is used to evaluate the aqueous component of the tear film and is valuable in the diagnosis of keratoconjunctivitis sicca (KCS) and other tear film abnormalities. The STT is indicated in all patients with external ocular disease. Individually wrapped sterile filter paper test strips may be dye impregnated to facilitate reading. Drops or manipulations should be avoided prior to STT; if there is discharge into and around the eye, dry cotton swabs should be used gently to clean the area, avoiding irritation and reflex lacrimation. The strips have a notch near one end where they are folded prior to use; fold the strip without touching it with the fingers, when it is still in the overwrap. Then open the package and, grasping the strip from the opposite end with fingers or forceps, place it into the lower conjunctival sac, approximately midway between the medial and lateral canthus, with the short folded end in the fornix and the notch on the lid margin. The lower lid can be rolled outward with the thumb to facilitate insertion, but care should be applied not to compress the eye, which may elicit reflex lacrimation. The lids may be maintained in an open position, or closed by gentle pressure on the upper lid if retention is a problem. After one minute, the moistened distance from the notch in the longer part is measured. Normal values in the dog are 15–25 mm min^{-1}; values less than 10 mm min^{-1} are highly suggestive of a deficit in aqueous tear production. Most of clinical cases of KCS have a wetting less than 5 mm min^{-1}. The cat has slightly lower and more variable normal values. There is a wide range of normalcy, and data should be interpreted in correlation with clinical signs. Increased production may be present if irritative processes are present.

Diagnostic stains

Fluorescein stain

Fluorescein is a water-soluble dye; owing to its lipid insolubility, it does not stain intact corneal epithelium, but does stain erosions or ulcers, which expose the hydrophilic stroma, allow penetration and retention of the dye. The barrier to penetration in the healthy eye resides in the outermost cells of the corneal epithelium. As Descemet's membrane does not retain fluorescein, descemetoceles will not stain. Fluorescein is available in the form of impregnated strips of paper or as a solution; the former are preferred because the solution may become contaminated with multiple usage. Individually wrapped strips ensure sterility and are preferred.

Fluorescein staining is indicated in all patients with ocular pain or observable corneal lesions. The fluorescein impregnated tip is moistened with a drop of sterile saline and the dorsal bulbar conjunctiva is gently touched. If the patient exhibits blepharospasm, local anesthetic can be instilled before the procedure or can be used instead of saline; it may cause a diffuse, slight positivity that is readily discernable from significant retention. Blinking will distribute the dye over the corneal surface. The excess dye is immediately flushed with a sterile saline solution rinse, which also enhances brightness of the dye. The eye is then examined with a focal light and magnification. A blue cobalt filter or a Wood's light will facilitate detection of subtle lesions. To evaluate nasolacrimal patency, apply the fluorescein as described above, but do not rinse the eye. If the ipsilateral nostril shows dye within 5 to 10 min, the nasolacrimal drainage system of that side is patent; the absence of dye passage, however, does not necessarily mean the contrary (see p. 213). Dye may be seen in the nasopharynx related to alternative duct openings, clinical implications are considered on p. 211 and 213.

Slit lamp observation of the fluorescein stained tear film while holding the lids open allows for evaluation of the tear break up time (BUT) as an indirect method of evaluating the non-aqueous components of the tear film (see p. 224); mucus deficiency will result in shortening of the BUT from the 20–30 s normally encountered. Test applications are elaborated on page 224.

Rose bengal

Rose bengal stains cells of the cornea and conjunctiva which are not covered by mucin; usually these are degenerating cells. The dye is available as a solution or impregnated strips; as with fluorescein, the latter are preferred. It may cause irritation which is worsened by light exposure. It is the preferred method for detecting dendritic intraepithelial erosions caused by herpesvirus, which may be difficult to detect with fluorescein, and in the detection of tear film abnormalities involving the lipid or mucin components of the tear film. Indications and application are identical to those described for fluorescein.

Cytology and culture

Cytology and culture of the conjunctiva and cornea are indicated in severe or chronic external ocular disease. Cells from the conjunctival fornix or the cornea may be harvested using a sterilized Kimura spatula, the blunt aspect of a sterile 64 surgical blade, or a cytologic brush. Sterile swabs wetted with sterile saline can also be used for this purpose, but usually will not provide as consistent results. Topical anesthesia can be used to facilitate collection and despite reports in the literature to the contrary in our experience does not significantly affect culture results. Collection of an adequate specimen requires firm but gentle pressure following irrigation to remove debris and secretions. It is important not to abrade or irritate the conjunctiva in order to avoid bleeding. The collected material may be placed directly into culture media and/or on a slide, concentrated in a small area to facilitate evaluation. Gram stain, Diff-Quik (Merze and Dade) and/or Giemsa are the routine stains of value. Unfixed and unstained slides may be submitted for or immunofluorescent antibody (IFA) studies. Biopsy material from feline conjunctiva or cornea may be sent for detection of the presence of herpesvirus, chlamydia, or other organisms by polymerase chain reaction (PCR).

Evaluation of the lacrimal drainage system

To evaluate the structure and function of the lacrimal puncta, lacrimal canaliculi, lacrimal sac, and nasolacrimal duct, topical anesthesia, sedation, or general anesthesia may be required in dogs, dependent on the nature of the patient. In cats, general anesthesia is usually required; the lacrimal puncta are smaller and less accessible. A curved stainless steel lacrimal cannula is preferred; 22–23 gauge works well in dogs, 26 gauge in cats. Its rigidity allows the operator to easily penetrate the bony opening of the lacrimal bone after having entered the lower punctum and nasolacrimal sac. The cannula should be mounted on a 2.5–3 ml syringe filled with sterile saline, or a small saline-filled compressible bottle.

The disadvantage of a rigid cannula is that of possible damage to the mucous membranes if the animal is not adequately restrained and anesthetized, or if the procedure is not gently performed. The cannula is inserted into the upper punctum, stretching the upper lid superiorly with the index finger to immobilize and straighten the canaliculus and facilitate cannula penetration. After the lacrimal punctum is entered, the system is flushed; saline will exit from the lower punctum. Then smooth movements are used to locate and enter the bony opening of the nasolacrimal duct. At this point, the lower punctum is closed with the thumb. The nasolacrimal duct is flushed and, keeping the nose of the animal angled downward, the fluid should flow from the ipsilateral nostril.

Direct ophthalmoscopy

The ophthalmoscope has a light source which is directed into the patient's eye so that the beam is nearly parallel with the line of sight of the examiner. A rheostat controls the light intensity while the dimension and the characteristics of the beam may be varied with a series of colored filters (the blue to excite fluorescein, the green to help differentiate pigment from retinal hemorrhage), a slit (to help evaluate the elevation of lesions), and a grid (to project onto the fundus in order to measure lesions). A selection of lenses ranging from + (black) 40 to −(red) 25 D (diopters) on a rotating wheel adjusts the depth of focus into the eye (Table 1.1). An accurate examination of the fundus of the eye can be performed only in a dark room through a well dilated pupil; 1–2 drops of 1% tropicamide should be applied at least 15–20 min prior to examination. Observation with a setting of around 0 to +1 or +2 D and the instrument held 1–2 feet from the eye provides critical evaluation of the fundus reflex, prior to observing the fundus from a distance of 1–2 inches and starting with a setting of 0, altered to achieve optimal focus. Direct ophthalmoscopy provides magnification of fundic features of 14 to 15 times. The disc is located and evaluated initially; the major vessels traced to the periphery, and each quadrant evaluated systematically to obtain a mental panorama. The main disadvantages of direct compared with indirect examination are the small field of vision, limited to about 4–5 mm of the fundus, and the risks due to the close proximity to the muzzle of uncooperative patients!

Hand lens monocular indirect ophthalmoscopy

The most economical way to perform indirect ophthalmoscopy is by using a 14–30 D hand lens and a focal light such as the Finoff transilluminator. Relatively expensive Nikon or Volk lenses or less inexpensive +10 to +20 magnifying lenses, 30–55 mm in diameter,

Table 2.1　Ophthalmoscope settings for examination of normal canine eyes

Structure	Ophthalmoscope settings (diopters)
Cornea	+15 to +20
Iris	+12 to +15
Anterior capsule of lens	+12 to +15
Posterior capsule of lens	+8 to +12
Vitreous	+2 to　+8
Optic disc and fundus	+2 to　−2

can be utilized. After dilation of the pupil and in a dark room, the observer should stand in front of the animal at arm's length, holding the transilluminator in front of the observer's own nose and the hand lens 5–6 cm in front of the patient's cornea (an assistant is required to restrain the patient's head and retract the lids). The fundus image should be made to fill the entire lens by moving the lens towards or away from the cornea.

Indentation tonometry

Tonometry is the assessment of intraocular pressure (IOP). Digital tonometry is a very crude technique; two-finger ballottement of the globe through the upper lids can detect a discrepancy between the two eyes, but should not be used without additional objective measurement. Instrumental tonometry may be performed by indentation or applanation. Indentation tonometry is based on the measurement of

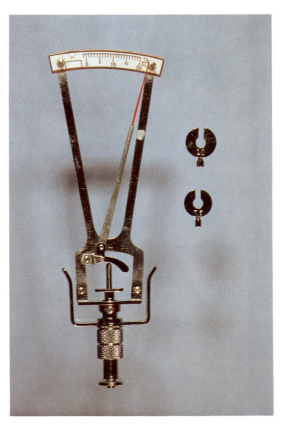

Figùre 2.1   A Schiøtz tonometer

the extent of indentation of the cornea obtained with a Schiøtz tonometer (Figure 2.1). It is a relatively inexpensive instrument which consists of a plunger which glides through a chamber stabilized by a bracket handle and which has a footplate which conforms with and is placed on the corneal surface. The plunger can be charged with different weights (5.5 g, 7.5 g, 10.0 g). Depending on how deeply the plunger indents the corneal surface, it moves a lever on the scale; this reading is converted to a value of IOP. Theoretically, the curvature and rigidity of the human cornea differ from that of the small animal cornea, so species-specific conversion tables are required for optimal quantitative accuracy; practically, indentation tonometry only estimates IOP and it is not critical if the table with human data that comes with the instrument or a veterinary scale is used. Normal values should be less than 25 mmHg. As a rule of thumb, scale values between 3 to 7 on the Schiøtz scale represent normal pressures in the dog, 2–6 in the cat, with the 5.5 g weight with readings less than 3 suggesting a raised IOP and those greater than 7 a hypotensive eye. Size of the eye (smaller eyes give values higher than actual IOP), age-related differences in scleral rigidity (young eyes are more elastic and give higher values as well), and corneal lesions can affect accuracy of results. Before each patient evaluation, the instrument should be calibrated on the convex steel test block; the indicator should read 0. The patient is given a few drops of topical anesthetic and the instrument is applied to the eye. Because the plunger is gravity driven, it is essential that the tonometer be held as close to perpendicular as possible and that its components are well cleaned and free moving. The footplate is applied to the cornea, elevating the head of the dog by the nose towards the ceiling. It is important not to occlude the jugular veins in order not to artifactually increase the IOP nor to compress the globe while retracting the eyelids, for the same reason. Occasionally it is easier to restrain a dog on its back, with the head held perpendicular to the body axis and the cornea in the horizontal plane. The measurement should be repeated several times in order to obtain three readings within 1–2 scale units of each other. The instrument should be placed as centrally as possible on the corneal surface, as the sclera has a different rigidity. The curved surface of the footplate should be in perfect and complete contact with the cornea. No force should be applied on the handle, which should be held gently to allow the instrument to rest freely on the corneal surface. Readings should be regarded as estimations of IOP rather than precise determinations. The main disadvantage is that the technique is demanding and requires practice to master.

Suggestions for reliable use include:

- Calibrate the tonometer before each use
- Ensure that the cornea is well anesthetized

- Most anesthetics and sedatives lower IOP (ketamine elevates)
- Do not compress the jugular veins or the globe
- Keep the cornea horizontal, the tonometer vertical and in the center of the cornea; avoid limbus and sclera as well as third eyelid (you can slip the footplate beneath the third eyelid if it protrudes)
- Make several measurements
- Always evaluate both eyes
- Consider breed and age variations
- Interpret readings in conjunction with other clinical signs
- After each use, dissemble and clean the instrument
- Make tonometry a part of your routine physical/ophthalmic examination to build confidence in your technique.

Instruments for more advanced diagnosis

To appreciate fully the anatomic details and pathologic changes of the eye, special examination techniques and more sophisticated equipment may be necessary to refine preliminary and differential diagnoses. While expense limits the availability of some of these instruments in general practice, they are an invaluable and essential tool for someone with a serious interest in ophthalmology.

Slit lamp

The slit lamp or biomicroscope allows precise localization of lesions within the adnexa, cornea, anterior chamber, lens, and anterior vitreous. These structures can be examined with high magnification; the beam of light can be shaped according to needs, either diffuse, or pinpoint (to detect subtle flare and cells), or a slit, and may be colored by inserting various filters. Observations of reflected and/or transmitted light provide a magnified three-dimensional view of the various optical structures.

Indirect ophthalmoscope

The monocular hand lens method, already described, can be replaced by a more sophisticated and expensive instrument, the monocular indirect ophthalmoscope, allowing an upright, wide angle view of the fundus. The more commonly used instrument is the binocular indirect ophthalmoscope which emits a bright light from a unit on the examiner's head which is directed into the eye of an animal; the emergent rays are converged by a 14–30 diopter convex condensing lens placed in the same fashion as in hand lens indirect ophthalmoscopy. The indirect method has several advantages over the direct one: both hands can be used to manipulate the patient's head and eyelids while the examiner is at arm's length from the animal; it is possible to obtain a panoramic view of the ocular fundus; and bright illumination can penetrate translucent ocular media. The disadvantages, compared with direct ophthalmoscopy, are the cost, the difficulty of mastering the technique, and the observation of a completely inverted and less magnified image ($\frac{1}{3}$ to $\frac{1}{4}$ that of the direct image). Systematic examination as described for direct ophthalmoscopy is recommended.

Applanation tonometry

In contrast to Schiøtz indentation tonometry, these tonometers measure the variable force necessary to flatten a constant small area of the cornea. The Tono Pen® (Figure 2.2) is a hand-held tonometer with several advantages over the Schiøtz tonometer, but is much more expensive. The stainless probe contains a solid state strain gauge

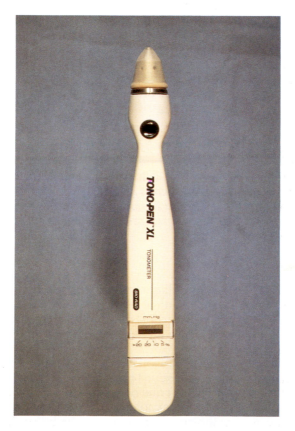

Figure 2.2   A Tono Pen® applanation tonometer

which converts intraocular pressure to an electrical signal. Every touch on the anesthetized cornea produces a waveform that is translated into a number on the digital display indicating the IOP expressed in mmHg. Every four valid readings, the device sounds a prolonged beep and the mean IOP is displayed. The tip probe of the instrument has to be covered with a disposable latex protective membrane to ensure sterility. The device is light and fits comfortably in the user's hand and can be used easily with any position of the animal's head, so minimal restraint is needed.

Gonioscopy

The iridocorneal angle is not directly visible without using a refractory lens placed on the corneal surface. In most cases, gonioscopy can be performed with topical anesthesia. Many different lenses are used in small animal ophthalmology with the Franklin, Barkan, and Koeppe lenses the most common; an indirect lens facilitates 360° examination simply by rotating the lens. The interface between lens and cornea is maintained with saline or 1.0% methylcellulose solutions. A coaxial light source and some magnification are needed for optimal observation (the biomicroscope is ideal); an otoscope can be satisfactorily used. The technique is indicated to evaluate glaucoma patients; when the glaucoma is unilateral, the presence of goniodysgenesis in the contralateral eye is an important risk factor as well as suggesting the pathogenesis of the glaucoma in the involved eye (see pp. 183).

Skiascopy (retinoscopy)

With this diagnostic procedure it is possible to evaluate an animal's refractive status, that is, to assess if an eye is emmetropic, myopic, or hyperopic. A hand held retinoscope with interposed positive and negative lenses is used to neutralize the movement of the observer's light source.

Ultrasonography

Ultrasound is a very helpful diagnostic procedure in ophthalmology. Two dimensional B-mode with a 10 MHz probe is ideal but very adequate studies can be performed with a 7.5 MHz probe which is available to practitioners who already use ultrasonography for other purposes.

The advantage of ocular ultrasonography is the ability to image the inner structures of the eye if lesions prevent direct observation. It also allows an evaluation of the soft and bony tissues of the orbit, making it of particular value in cases of exophthalmos and proptosis. Suspected intraocular disease in the presence of opaque media, uveal neoplasia, and orbital diseases are the major indications for ultrasound.

Radiology

Radiology is used in small animal ophthalmology as a preliminary for other imaging techniques (ultrasound, CAT scan, MRI), which generally provide more information. Orbital bone, sinus, and skull evaluation are the main indications. Dacryocystorhinography allows evaluation of the nasolacrimal duct.

Computerized Axial Tomography (CAT)

A CAT scan is recommended when critical evaluation of the orbit is required. Detailed imaging of the orbital contents, including globe, extraocular muscles, and optic nerve, as well as the adjacent bony skull and sinuses, is invaluable in the diagnosis of orbital neoplastic, inflammatory, or traumatic disease.

Magnetic Resonance Imaging

Magnetic resonance imaging (MRI) offers enhanced projection and resolution of soft tissues compared with a CAT scan and is of particular value in neurophthalmology.

Electroretinography (ERG) and visual evoked response (VER)

The ERG records the mass response of the retina to light stimulus through surface electrodes at the cornea and at the lateral canthus. The VER simultaneously records the activity of the visual cortex. Two main waves characterize the ERG:

- The initial negative *a*-wave is thought to arise from the inner segments of photoreceptors (rods and cones)
- The following positive *b*-wave is thought to arise from the inner nuclear layer and possibly from the Müller cells.

In addition to the *a*- and *b*- waves, there is usually a second positive deflection, the *c*-wave, which is more prolonged and probably arises from the retinal pigment epithelium.

Electrophysiology is indicated when critical assessment of the afferent visual components and pathways is required and may be a more sensitive indicator of retinal health than ophthalmoscopy. Differentiation between external and more central causes of visual impairment may also be accomplished.

Fluorescein angiography

The ocular vascular system and the integrity of the blood ocular barriers can be observed by direct ophthalmoscopy using an exciting wavelength of light (blue) and the appropriate filters (yellow) following the intravenous injection of fluorescein dye. The technique is useful to evaluate neovascular or inflammatory changes.

EXAMINATION OF THE EYE

The first step to ophthalmic diagnosis is to collect a thorough history; while doing this, the animal should be left free to move about the room, so that a first impression of alertness, visual acuity, and behavior is registered. Ocular examination should be conducted routinely as a part of the general physical examination. A systematic standard approach is suggested for a quick but complete eye examination, first in ambient light, then in a dark room (Figure 2.3).

Light room examination

This consists of evaluating the gross appearance of eye and surrounding structures to determine the presence of periorbital swelling, lacrimation, or abnormal discharge, and the size and position of the eye. Examination of the anterior segment of the eye follows. Both eyes must always be considered, even if only one is obviously affected. In such instances it is better to examine the normal eye first. The magnification loupe and focal illumination are used to assess the adnexa and anterior segment structures. The STT, if indicated, is performed before additional manipulations or applications are performed.

PLR, menace response, blinking, and ocular, and periocular sensation should then be evaluated. PLR can be tested in ambient light; repeat the procedure in a darkened room if abnormalities are noted. First each eye is directly stimulated with a bright focal light and the completeness and briskness of the PLR is noted. This is the direct reflex, while the pupil of the opposite eye constricts due to the consensual reflex. For anatomical reasons in non-primates, the consensual pupil may not constrict to exactly the same size as the pupil of the stimulated eye. The menace reflex should be tested next, paying attention not to cause air movement toward the patient's eye and a consequent blink (mediated by the trigeminal nerve). Bear in mind that the absence of the menace reflex is normal in very young animals.

Critically evaluate globe size and position, palpate around the orbital rim and retropulse both globes simultaneously. Distinction

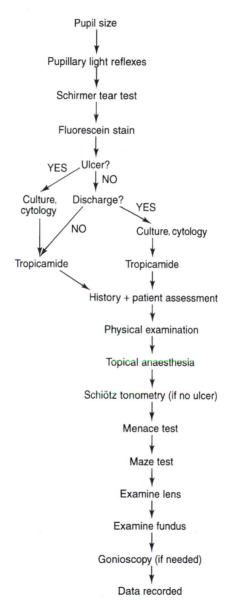

Figure 2.3 Flowchart for ophthalmic examination.

between exophthalmus and globe enlargement is critical. Then consider the eyelids, third eyelid, conjunctiva, sclera, cornea, and anterior chamber, iris, lens and anterior vitreous, one by one, using the magnification loupe and the focal light. If the adnexa is inflamed and there is discharge, STT is indicated, and cytology and culture should be considered. If a serous discharge is bilateral without evidence of inflammation, or the discharge is concentrated on the medial aspect and the hyperemia is particularly evident in the medial canthus, the lacrimal drainage system should be investigated, with a suspicion of obstruction and/or dacryocystitis. If the patient exhibits blepharospasm, look for corneal ulcers, a foreign body, entropion, or ectopic cilia, and stain with fluorescein. Chronic disorders of the cornea manifested by neovascularization and melanosis may be associated with trichiasis, distichiasis, lagophthalmos, lacrimal secretory disorders, or immune-mediated disease. If intraocular disease is suspected, based on the presence of episcleral/scleral injection, corneal edema, aqueous cells or flare, or abnormal PLRs, tonometry is a requisite. Congestion of episcleral vessels may be differentiated from conjunctival injection by applying one drop of phenylephrine; in cases of conjunctivitis the hyperemic pattern will almost completely disappear. Uveitis also must be considered in case of a red eye. Because pupillary dilatation is necessary for the remainder of the ophthalmic exam, one drop of 1.0% tropicamide should be applied to each eye at this point (perform the rest of the general physical examination in the interim).

Dark room examination

When the pupils are completely dilated as an effect of the previously instilled mydriatic, the lens, vitreous, and the ocular fundus may be carefully examined. The lens can be examined by moving the transilluminator to the right and to the left from the frontal position in such a way as to shift the incidental light and better visualize any opacity with the magnification loupe. By inserting the positive lenses of the direct ophthalmoscope between +8 and +12, as described in Table 2.1, it is then possible to localize the opacity with a certain approximation. The fundus should be evaluated using the indirect or direct ophthalmoscope.

Gonioscopy is not often performed by the general practitioner, but if it is needed, it is preferable to perform it prior to mydriasis.

During all steps of the examination, all data should be recorded in the patient's permanent record and, in case of consultation, transmitted to the veterinary ophthalmologist.

3

THERAPEUTICS

Bruce H Grahn and Joe Wolfer

INTRODUCTION

The eye is a delicate and complex organ which is affected by a variety of diseases. Successful medical management of ocular disease is based not only on an accurate diagnosis but also in-depth knowledge of pharmacology. The purpose of this chapter is to enhance the veterinarian's understanding of ocular therapeutics by reviewing the pharmacokinetics and indications for topical, subconjunctival, and systemic drugs that are commonly prescribed for diseases of the eye.

The eye may be medicated topically, systemically, or by injection into the subconjunctival, intraocular, or orbital spaces. There are several compartments in the eye, separated by semi-permeable barriers. The cornea is normally avascular which limits delivery of systemic medications via the circulatory system with the exception of those agents secreted in the tears. Topical or subconjunctival medications are appropriate for most corneal diseases. Diseases of the anterior segment may be medicated topically, subconjunctivally, or systemically, while most posterior segment, orbit, and eyelid diseases require systemic medications. As intraocular and intraorbital injections have inherent risks and should be performed by an ophthalmologist, they will not be described in this chapter. When an animal is to be medicated at home, owner compliance is an important and often forgotten factor. The owner must have the time and ability to medicate the eye during the specified treatment period and the knowledge of what to expect in terms of improvement or deterioration in the condition. Treatment instructions should be given to the owner verbally and in written form. Consider the following with regard to owner compliance. Topical solutions are usually easier to apply than ointments but they require more frequent application. Is the animal manageable by the owner alone and if not will an assistant be available to restrain the animal during medication? Will painful orbital or ocular inflammation preclude administration of medications? If the medications are used for an extended period of time, has the most economical formulation been selected?

PHARMACOKINETICS OF OPHTHALMIC DRUGS

The clinician should have a basic understanding of the pharmacokinetics of topical, subconjunctival, and systemic ophthalmic drugs. The most frequently used route for ocular therapy is topical. The availability of a topical medication for the eye is principally dependent on the drug concentration and kinetics in the conjunctival cul-de-sac, corneal permeability, and the rate of elimination of the medication from the conjunctival sac [1]. Tear flow and space within the conjunctival fornix have a dynamic effect on topical ophthalmic medications. Commercial droppers deliver 25–50 µl/drop of solution or suspension and immediate reflex tearing occurs after a drop of medication is placed on the eye. The non-blinking eye will retain approximately 10–25 µl (varies with species) of additional fluid in the conjunctival fornix and tear film, after which immediate overflow occurs [2]. Application of more than one drop at a time will not increase the amount of available drug because this volume and the reflex tears will overflow into the nasolacrimal duct or onto the eyelid [3]. It is important to wait 5 min between application of consecutive topical medications. Only 20% of the medication will remain on the ocular surface after 5 min [2]. This rapid reduction is the result of drainage through the nasolacrimal system and absorption of the medication through the cornea and conjunctiva. Most of the intraocular penetration of topically applied medications occurs via the cornea [4]. The cornea has a thick hydrophilic stroma which is enveloped by two thin lipophilic structures, the epithelium and endothelium. Drug factors such as solubility, ionization, and molecular size affect absorption. Membrane factors including weakness or absence of portions of the cornea are also important [5]. The stroma is a significant barrier for lipophilic drugs which consequently accumulate in the epithelium. The epithelium is a significant barrier for hydrophilic drugs. In order to penetrate the cornea well, drugs require both hydrophilic and lipophilic characteristics.

Topical ophthalmic drugs are available as solutions, emulsions, and ointments. Emulsions and ointments have slightly prolonged contact times compared to solutions and therefore require less frequent administration. However, emulsions have the disadvantage of being less stable and ointments are more difficult to apply and elicit rubbing and pawing. For a further review of pharmacokinetics and corneal penetration of topically applied ophthalmic drugs, the reader is referred to Shell [6] and Burstein and Anderson[7].

Subconjunctival injection of medications can be a valuable adjunct to topical therapy if the practitioner understands the indications and limitations of the use of the injection. Medications, including some of the antibiotics, enjoy enhanced ocular penetration with bulbar subconjunctival injections [8]. In fractious or aggressive patients, subconjunctival injection under sedation may be the only means of therapy.

The pharmacokinetics of subconjunctival injections is poorly understood and likely varies considerably between classes of drugs and their formulations. Medications injected into the subconjunctival space are thought to enter the ciliary circulation thereby gaining access to the anterior segment. However, some of the drug simply leaks through the puncture site in the conjunctiva and is absorbed directly through the cornea [9]. In the case of subconjunctival corticosteroids, penetration of the sclera has also been reported [10]. Direct absorption of medication from the injection site bypasses the epithelial barrier and increases intraocular drug availability by avoiding tear dilution [11]. The use of subconjunctival medications at surgery minimizes the need for topical medications during the immediate postoperative period. Other advantages include increased intraocular concentration of drugs that penetrate the cornea poorly, and ensured drug application when the owner compliance is poor [12].

Subconjunctival injections require the utmost care. Topical anesthesia is required and occasionally sedation or general anesthesia is necessary to ensure accurate bulbar subconjunctival injection. A subconjunctival injection is performed by gently grasping the dorsal bulbar conjunctiva with small tissue forceps (i.e. Bishop Harmon). A 25 gauge needle (attached to a 1 ml syringe) is inserted bevel up through the tented bulbar conjunctiva. Up to 0.5 ml of medication may be slowly injected to form a subconjunctival bleb. The dosage will vary with the ocular condition and medication but the total volume per injection site should not exceed 0.5 ml. Long lasting [depot] medications should be avoided as they are irritating and may predispose to granuloma formation [13]. Subconjunctival injections of solutions including antibiotics and atropine need to be repeated every 24 hr. The repetition rate will vary depending on the response to therapy and the frequency of topical and systemic medications. Subconjunctival injections of long lasting steroids, i.e. betamethasone valerate, need to be repeated every 7–10 days.

There are inherent risks associated with the use of subconjunctival injections. Complications include irritation at the injection site, granuloma formation, inadvertent intraocular injections, and an inability to withdraw medications if necessary. Some medications are too irritating and should not be administered subconjunctivally.

Systemic medications may be administered orally, intramuscularly, intravenously, or subcutaneously for therapy of glaucoma, and eyelid, orbital, posterior segment, and optic nerve diseases. Systemic antibiotics, corticosteroids, non-steroidal anti-inflammatory drugs

(NSAIDs) and carbonic anhydrase inhibitors are commonly administered for these conditions. The blood ocular barrier is composed of tight junctions of the endothelium of the iris and retinal blood vessels and the cillary and retinal pigment epithelium. This barrier is only penetrated by a few lipophilic drugs of low molecular weight (e.g. chloramphenicol). However with inflammatory eye conditions the blood ocular barrier is disrupted, which allows most systemic medications to accumulate in the anterior and posterior segments. Antibiotics should be selected initially on the basis of cytologic evaluation of fine needle aspirates from the eye, eyelid, or orbit and are re-evaluated when bacterial cultures and sensitivities are available. Systemic corticosteroids are indicated in most inflammatory conditions of the posterior segment except when cornea ulceration is present. Prednisone, prednisolone, dexamethasone, or flumethasone are common choices for severe posterior segment, optic nerve or orbital inflammation. Systemic NSAIDs are frequently administered to control inflammation of the posterior segment or orbit. Examples include flunixin, aspirin, ketoprofen and indomethacin. Contraindications for NSAIDs include platelet disorders, coagulopathies, and specific hypersensitivities to these drugs. Systemic carbonic anhydrase inhibitors decrease the production of aqueous humor by the non-pigmented ciliary epithelium and are indicated for treatment of acute glaucoma and prophylactic treatment of primary glaucoma. Examples of these include dichlorophenamide and acetazolamide. These medications are contraindicated when acidosis or hypokalemia are present as they will aggravate these conditions. Clinical manifestations of acidosis and hypokalemia include panting, vomiting, diarrhea, and collapse.

Numerous fixed ratio topical ophthalmic medications are available and frequently prescribed by veterinarians. It is our opinion that these medications (usually an antibiotic and steroid combination) are over used, often because of a lack of a specific diagnosis. Topical or systemic corticosteroid therapy does not require the addition of antibiotics and vice versa. If both are required for separate purposes then separate formulations are usually more appropriate to deliver adequate concentrations of each.

ANTIMICROBIALS

Topical antimicrobials (antibiotics, antifungals, and antivirals)

Topical antibiotics may be categorized, based on their intended use, into primary, secondary and tertiary types. Primary antibiotics are used to treat bacterial conjunctivitis and simple corneal ulcers. The bacterial flora of the dog and cat ocular surface are a mixed population of predominantly Gram-positive organisms [14, 15]. Therefore, broad spectrum antibiotics including triple antibiotics (neomycin, polymyxin B, bacitracin), gentamicin, or chloramphenicol are appropriate for conjunctivitis or simple corneal ulcers. Triple antibiotics and gentamicin are bactericidal. Chloramphenicol is bacteriostatic but penetrates the eye rapidly and achieves high intraocular concentrations. Secondary level antibiotics are selected for specific anterior segment conditions. An example is tetracycline, which is the antibiotic of choice for feline *Chlamydia* or *Mycoplasma* conjunctivitis. It is bacteriostatic and achieves an adequate concentration in the cornea and conjunctiva. Tertiary level antibiotics should be reserved for severe infectious conditions including melting corneal ulcers and panophthalmitis. An example is tobramycin, an aminoglycoside which is bactericidal and effective against most Gram-negative bacteria including *Pseudomonas.*

Bacterial infections of the cornea or anterior segment require a minimum of one drop QID therapy with antibiotic solutions or emulsions for 7 days or until the infection is resolved. When ointments are prescribed, a 5 mm strip is applied to the conjunctiva, a minimum of three times per day until the infection is resolved. Ointments are contraindicated when the cornea is perforated because they are very irritating to the uvea [3]. Topical gentamicin should be avoided when the cornea is perforated. Toxic effects on the corneal endothelium and the retina and ciliary epithelium have been reported when those tissues were exposed to high concentrations of gentamicin [16, 17].

Idoxuridine, adenine arabinoside, and trifluridine are topical antivirals that have been used to treat feline herpetic keratitis and conjunctivitis. Idoxuridine mimics thymidine, thereby altering virus metabolism. It is available as a solution or ointment and should be applied frequently (q2hr for 2 weeks) and q6hr for 4 weeks. Adenine arabinoside inhibits virus DNA polymerase. It is available as an ointment and should be applied q4hr for several weeks to be effective. Trifluridine inhibits viral DNA synthesis and is available as a solution which is applied q4hr for at least 3 weeks. Trifluridine has the highest *in vitro* activity against feline herpesvirus. Herpetic keratitis and conjunctivitis are difficult to control and the search for an effective topical antiviral is ongoing.

Fungal infections of the dog and cat eye are uncommon and are usually limited to the cornea. They are difficult to treat and referral to an ophthalmologist and treatment with topical antifungal ophthalmic medications including natamycin, miconazole, clotrimazole, silver sulfadiazine, or povidone-iodine may be required. Natamycin is the only available commercial topical ophthalmic antifungal. It is available as a solution which should be administered q6hr until the corneal fungal infection is eliminated. Miconazole solutions may be administered topically or subconjunctivally. Clotrimazole and silver sulfadiazine are available as dermatologic ointments which may be applied topically on the eye [18]. Dilute povidone-iodine solution has also been reported as a topical ophthalmic antifungal agent [18].

Subconjunctival antimicrobials

Antibiotic or antifungal solutions may be injected under the bulbar conjunctiva as adjunct therapy for bacterial or fungal infections of the anterior segment. Medications inadvertently placed under the palpebral conjunctiva are not considered as useful since the blood circulation is away from the eye in this location. Gentamicin, penicillin, or cephalosporins are appropriate antibiotics for subconjunctival injections. Miconazole solution can be administered as an antifungal agent. These injections increase the anterior segment concentration of the drug by absorption into the anterior ciliary circulation and by drainage over the cornea from the injection site. The contraindications for these forms of therapy include known hypersensitivities. Conjunctival and episcleral irritation are commonly observed with this form of therapy.

Systemic antimicrobials

Bacterial infections of the eyelid, orbit, and uvea require systemic antibiotic therapy. Ideally these antibiotics are chosen on the basis of culture and sensitivity results. However these are seldom available at the critical stage of early infection. Cytologic evaluations of fine needle aspirates from the infected intraocular or orbital contents should be performed when aerobic and anaerobic cultures are collected. Cytology will often aid the clinician in identification of the potential bacteria and in selection of an appropriate antibiotic. Bactericidal antibiotics that are effective against aerobic and anaerobic bacteria are appropriate for most of these infections. Beta-lactams including ampicillin, amoxicillin, or cephalosporins are recommended and they are available in oral, intravenous, intramuscular, and subcutaneous forms. The antibiotic selected should be reconsidered after cultures and sensitivities are available. The visual prognosis is often dependent on prompt control of intraocular or orbital infections. Intravenous therapy is recommended to establish immediate tissue concentrations. Intramuscular or oral therapy should be continued until the clinical signs of the infection are gone. Most systemic antibiotics will penetrate infected intraocular tissues because the blood ocular barrier has been broken.

Systemic antifungals (i.e. amphotericin B, ketoconazole, flucytosine, itraconazole, thiabendazole) have been reported in the therapy of blastomycosis, coccidioidomycosis, cryptococcosis, and histoplasmosis. For a review of the systemic antifungal therapy of ocular and systemic mycosis, the reader is referred to Noxon *et al.* [19].

Acyclovir is a systemic antiviral drug that has been administered to cats with herpesvirus, conjunctivitis, and keratitis. Acyclovir is a thymidine kinase substrate which interferes with viral DNA synthesis. This medication is administered orally at a dose of 2 mg/kg for 21 days. The effectiveness of this medication against feline herpes is controversial [20, 21].

ANTI-INFLAMMATORY MEDICATIONS

Topical anti-inflammatories

Topical corticosteroids and NSAIDs are commonly used to control inflammation of the anterior segment. Corticosteroids and NSAIDs may be used in combination for severe intraocular inflammation.

Topical ophthalmic corticosteroids

Corticosteroids inhibit phospholipase which alters the arachidonic acid metabolic pathway and minimizes inflammation. Corticosteroids decrease vasodilation, capillary permeability, leukocyte infiltration, and release of inflammatory mediators from cells. They also inhibit fibroblasts and collagen formation. Corticosteroids are available in several forms. The acetate forms are more lipophilic which allows for better corneal penetration when compared to succinates or phosphates. Dexamethasone and prednisone are excellent selections for control of anterior segment inflammation. They are available as suspensions or ointments. Topical corticosteroids are contraindicated when corneal ulceration is present. Continuous topical corticosteroid therapy will induce adrenal gland suppression.

Topical NSAIDs

These drugs inhibit the cyclo-oxygenase pathway and reduce intraocular inflammation. Their inhibition of cyclo-oxygenase and endoperoxide isomerase enzymes decreases the production of prostaglandins, which cause miosis, altered blood aqueous barrier, vasodilation, and increased vascular permeability. Topical ophthalmic NSAIDs are indicated to control most anterior segment inflammation. There are several topical ophthalmic NSAIDs available including flurbiprofen, ketoralac, diclofenac, and profenal. They should be used with caution when corneal ulceration is present as delayed epithelial healing may occur. Topical NSAIDs are contraindicated in animals with glaucoma as they may increase the intraocular pressure. They should be avoided or used with caution in animals with platelet dyscrasias as they may decrease platelet aggregation and promote intraocular hemorrhage.

Topical mast cell stabilizers and antihistamines

Cromolyn sodium solution is a topical mast cell stabilizer which prevents the release of inflammatory mediators from mast cells. It is useful in the treatment of inflammatory conjunctival diseases where mast cells predominate, such as allergic conjunctivitis. Several topical human antihistamines are available commercially including antazoline, pheniramine maleate and pyrilamine. They are useful if applied during the acute stages of allergic conjunctivitis.

Subconjunctival anti-inflammatory drugs

Subconjunctival corticosteroids are indicated to control progressive, poorly responsive anterior segment inflammation. They provide antiinflammatory effects to the anterior segment via the ciliary circulation, and by seepage of the medication onto the cornea through the bulbar conjunctival injection site. Subconjunctival corticosteroid injections are contraindicated when corneal ulceration is present. Conjunctival and episcleral inflammation and granulomas occur frequently after long acting corticosteroid injections and their usage should be discouraged. Prednisone, dexamethasone, or betamethasone sodium phosphate may be recommended as adjunctive therapy for non-responsive immune-mediated anterior segment inflammation.

Systemic anti-inflammatories

Systemic corticosteroids may be required to control severe anterior and posterior segment inflammation. Similar to antibiotics they readily concentrate intraocularly when the blood ocular barrier has been broken. They are contraindicated when corneal ulcers are present as they delay epithelization and healing. Prednisone and dexamethasone are the most frequently prescribed. They may be administered orally, subcutaneously, intramuscularly, or intravenously at immune suppressive doses for prednisone (2 mg/kg) and dexamethasone (0.5 mg/kg) or anti-inflammatory doses for prednisone (1mg/kg) and dexamethasone (0.125 mg/kg) in the dog and cat.

The commonly used systemic NSAIDs include flunixin meglumine, aspirin, and ketoprofen. They may be administered intravenously (flunixin meglumine) or orally (aspirin, ketoprofen). Flunixin meglumine is often administered to dogs prior to intraocular surgery. It should not be administered for longer than 3 days [22]. Aspirin or ketoprofen may be administered to control intraocular inflammation.

The recommended dosage for aspirin is 10 mg/kg BID in the dog and 10 mg/kg q 72–96 hr in the cat. The recommended dosage for ketoprofen in the dog and cat is 1 mg/kg q24 hr. Systemic NSAIDs are contraindicated in patients with bleeding disorders, impaired renal function, or pre-existing hypersensitivities and they predispose the animal to gastrointestinal ulceration.

OCULAR HYPOTENSIVE DRUGS

These drugs lower the intraocular pressure by reducing the rate of production of aqueous humor, by increasing the rate of outflow of aqueous humor, or via a combination of these actions. They are useful in the emergency management of acute glaucoma, as adjunctive medical therapy to surgical procedures, and as prophylactic medications to slow the onset of primary glaucoma. They are available in topical and systemic formulations.

Topical ocular hypotensive drugs

Parasympathomimetics

Parasympathomimetics may be direct acting (i.e. have their effect directly on cholinergic receptors) or be indirect acting and inhibit acetylcholinesterase. These medications lower the intraocular pressure by altering the filtration angle which increases the outflow of aqueous humor.

Direct acting parasympathomimetics

Pilocarpine is a parasympathomimetic that is commonly used to lower the intraocular pressure. Pilocarpine is a potent miotic and is available as a solution or gel. Pilocarpine should be administered 3–4 times/day and it is frequently used in combination with other anti-glaucoma drugs including beta-adrenergic blockers, adrenergics, and systemic carbonic anhydrase inhibitors. Pilocarpine is contraindicated in uveitis and secondary glaucoma because of its miotic effects which may predispose to posterior synechiae and pupillary occlusion. A frequently observed side effect is a conjunctival hypersensitivity after prolonged use. This hypersensitivity warrants dilution of the pilocarpine or discontinuance of this drug.

Indirect acting parasympathomimetics

Cholinesterase inhibitors are categorized into reversible and irreversible agents. Physostigmine salicylate is a reversible cholinesterase inhibitor with a short duration of activity which limits its use to a diagnostic agent for parasympathetic disorders. Demecarium bromide is an irreversible carbamate inhibitor that is available as a topical solution. It is a potent cholinesterase inhibitor that lowers the intraocular pressure and has a duration of action of approximately 12–48 hr. Isoflurophate and echothiophate iodide are irreversible cholinesterase inhibitors. They are also long acting, potent organophosphate drugs that lower the intraocular pressure. They are administered on a 12–48 hr basis in the dog.

Parasympthomimetics are often directly irritating to the eye and may produce painful spasms of the ciliary and iridial muscles. Systemic toxicity may also develop and the clinical signs include salivation, vomiting, diarrhea, and abdominal cramps. These drugs should be used with caution and avoided when systemic anticholinesterases are being administered.

Adrenergics

Epinephrine and dipivefrin are adrenergic agents that lower the intraocular pressure in the dog and cat. Their mechanism of action is not completely understood, however the outflow facility has been shown to increase and the aqueous humor formation may decrease [23]. Epinephrine and dipivefrine solutions are administered q8hrs. Contraindications include known sensitivities to adrenergic medications and predisposition to arrhythmias.

Alpha-adrenergic agonist

Alpha-adrenergic agonists notably aproclonidine hydrochloride lower IOP by decreasing aqueous production in humans and rabbits; the effect is transient and a 1·0% solution may be of value in the dog in managing the IOP elevations that may occur following surgical procedures, including cataract extraction and cyclocryosurgery.

Adrenergic antagonists

Numerous topical adrenergic antagonists are available for treating glaucoma. Very few of these agents have been critically evaluated in the dog or cat. The beta-blocker timolol maleate has been shown to reduce the aqueous humor production in the dog significantly [24], and in the cat by up to 71% [25]. Timolol decreases the rate of aqueous humor production by reduction of blood flow through the ciliary processes. It is available as a solution and may be administered topically, one drop q12hr in dogs and cats. These drugs are contraindicated in animals with known sensitivities to beta-blockers including some cardiovascular and respiratory diseases.

Carbonic anhydrase inhibitors

A topical carbonic anhydrase inhibitor, dorzolamide hydrochloride, is now available. It is too early to judge its efficacy in the management of glaucoma in companion animals. A 2% solution is applied q8hrs. Topical application should avoid the potential side effects associated with this class of drugs.

Systemic ocular hypotensive medications

Systemic medications that reduce intraocular pressure include carbonic anhydrase inhibitors, mannitol, and glycerine. Carbonic anhydrase inhibitors reduce the intraocular pressure by decreasing the rate of aqueous humor production. Examples of carbonic anhydrase inhibitors include dichlorophenamide, acetazolamide, and methazolamide. Dichlorophenamide is currently the carbonic anhydrase of choice as it effectively lowers the intraocular pressure and has the least side effects. Carbonic anhydrase inhibitors are contraindicated in dogs or cats with a predisposition to or concurrent acidosis. Topical carbonic anhydrase inhibitors are now available and are aimed at avoiding the systemic side effects of these drugs.

Intravenous mannitol solution and oral glycerine paste reduce the vitreous volume by osmosis and lower the intraocular pressure. They are indicated in the emergency management of canine glaucoma. Water should be restricted for 1 hr after administration to attain maximum effect. Glycerine is contraindicated in the vomiting patient and both are contraindicated in patients with congestive heart failure, hypertension, or renal failure [26]. Their use in the diabetic patient is controversial [3, 26, 27].

MYDRIATICS AND CYCLOPLEGICS

Mydriasis is dilation of the pupil, and cycloplegia is paralysis of the ciliary muscle which results in a loss of accommodative function. Parasympatholytics paralyse the iris sphincter muscle and cause mydriasis. Cycloplegia may develop depending on the type of parasympatholytic administered. Sympathomimetics stimulate the adrenergic receptors of the dilator muscle and may cause mydriasis.

Parasympatholytics

Tropicamide is available as a topical ophthalmic solution. Tropicamide has minimal effect on the ciliary muscles, has a rapid onset of action (20 min), is short acting (3–4 hr) and it is the mydriatic of choice for intraocular examinations. Atropine has a slow onset of action (45 min) and the pupillary dilatation is accompanied by cycloplegia. Atropine is available as a topical ophthalmic solution or ointment and as a systemic medication which can be administered subconjunctivally. Topical or subconjunctival atropine are recommended for mydriasis and cycloplegia in uveitis in the dog and cat. Atropine may be required as often as every 6 hr to maintain comfort by control of the ciliary spasm or as needed on a daily basis when the uveitis is minimal. Mild to moderate salivation is a common side effect of these drugs as they are bitter tasting, reaching the mouth via drainage through the nasolacrimal duct. Systemic side effects of atropine include tachycardia and decreased gastrointestinal motility.

Sympathomimetics

Phenylephrine and epinephrine are examples of sympathomimetics. They are available as topical ophthalmic solutions which have a synergistic effect with parasympatholytics. This synergistic activity is useful in cases of miosis associated with severe uveitis. Dilute solutions of epinephrine and phenylephrine may be useful for differentiation of pre- and post-ganglionic Horner's syndrome. Intracameral injections of sterile dilute solutions of epinephrine or phenylephrine are also administered during intraocular surgery to maintain mydriasis and control capillary bleeding. Adrenergics are contraindicated in patients with a predisposition to cardiac arrhythmias or known sensitivities to these drugs.

Indirect acting sympathomimetics

Cocaine and hydroxyamphetamine are indirect acting sympathomimetics which are administered topically to differentiate pre- and post-ganglionic Horner's syndrome. Hydroxyamphetamine is reported to be the drug of choice for differentiation of central and pre-ganglionic from post-ganglionic Horner's syndrome [28]. However the availability and need for strict control of these potentially addictive drugs has limited their use in veterinary medicine.

LACRIMOMIMETIC DRUGS AND ARTIFICIAL TEARS

Cyclosporine is a potent immunosuppressive drug that is very useful in the treatment of immune mediated keratoconjunctivitis sicca (KCS) in the dog. It is a T-cell suppressor which decreases lacrimal gland inflammation. In addition this drug has a direct lacrimomimetic effect and it also reduces corneal inflammation. It is available commercially as a 0.2% ophthalmic ointment and has been compounded as a 1% and 2% solution and as a 1% emulsion. A quarter of an inch strip of the ointment is applied to the cornea every 12 hr. If instituted early in the course of immune-mediated keratoconjunctivitis sicca, topical cyclosporine will reverse the low tear production and the Schirmer tear test will usually return to normal within 6 weeks. Topical cyclosporine is poorly absorbed through the cornea and has minimal systemic effects. It may be used when corneal ulcers are present and it remains the drug of choice for dry eye in the dog [29]. In addition it has been reported as an effective agent in the control of chronic superficial keratitis in the dog [30]. The contraindications for topical ophthalmic cyclosporine include keratomycosis and known hypersensitivities to cyclosporine or its carriers.

Pilocarpine has been reported to be an effective lacrimomimetic drug in the treatment of neurogenic KCS [31]. Oral pilocarpine can be toxic and should be administered with caution to dogs. Signs of toxicity include vomiting and diarrhea. If these signs present, the drug should be discontinued.

Tear replacements

Numerous tear supplements are available. These include hypertonic, isotonic, and hypotonic tear solutions. In addition, tear replacements are available as ointments which provide a longer duration of effect compared to the solutions. Artificial tears, hydroxymethylcellulose, and polyvinyl alcohols should be administered frequently and are usually required in excess of q4hr to prevent corneal dehydration. Hyaluronic acid solutions increase the duration of tear contact and stabilize the tear film and they are useful adjunctive agents in the treatment of qualitative and quantitative tear film abnormalities in the dog and cat.

MISCELLANEOUS TOPICAL DRUGS

Proparacaine and tetracaine are topical anesthetics that are required prior to tonometry and to facilitate the ocular examination. Topical anesthetics are toxic to the corneal epithelium and repetitive or prolonged use is strongly discouraged as it may lead to severe corneal ulceration, or even perforation. The preservatives that are present are reported to interfere with bacterial cultures [32]. Ideally laboratory submissions including bacterial, fungal and viral cultures, and cytologic samples should be collected prior to application any topical solutions, emulsions, or ointments.

Fluorescein and rose bengal are stains which are routinely used in ocular examinations. Fluorescein is a water-soluble dye which readily penetrates the conjunctival submucosa or the corneal stroma when the lipophilic epithelium has been disrupted. It is applied topically during the ophthalmic examination to confirm corneal ulceration. It is available as an impregnated strip or solution. Rose bengal is available as an impregnated strip. It is a supravital dye that is used to detect devitalized epithelium. These stains will interfere with bacterial and viral cultures and immunocytology and therefore those laboratory submissions should be completed before these stains are applied [33, 34].

REFERENCES

1. Mishima S. Clinical pharmacokinetics of the eye. *Invest. Ophthalmol. Vis. Sci.* 1981; **21**: 504–41.
2. Peiffer RL and Stowe CM. Veterinary ophthalmic pharmacology. In: Gelatt KN (ed) *Veterinary Ophthalmology*, Philadelphia: Lea & Febiger 1981: 160–205.
3. Regnier A and Toutain PL. Ocular pharmacology and therapeutic modalities. In: Gelatt KN (ed). *Veterinary Ophthalmology*, 2nd edn. Philadelphia: Lea & Febiger 1991: 162–94.
4. Doane MG, Jensen AD and Dohlman CH. Penetration routes of topically applied eye medications. *Am. J. Ophthalmol.* 1978; **85**: 383.
5. Schoenwald RD. Ocular drug delivery. Pharmacokinetic considerations. *Clin. Pharmacokinet.* 1990; **18**: 255–69.
6. Shell JW. Pharmacokinetics of topically applied ophthalmic drugs. *Surv. Ophthalmol.* 1982; **26**: 207–18.
7. Burstein NL and Anderson JA. Review: Corneal penetration and ocular bioavailability of drugs. *J. Ocular Pharmacol.* 1985; **1**: 309–26.
8. Bartlett JD and Cullen AP. Clinical administration of ocular drugs. In: Barlett JD and Jaanus SD (eds) *Clinical Ocular Pharmacology*, Toronto: Butterworth-Heinemann 1989: 29–66.
9. Wine NA, Gonall AG and Basu PK. The ocular uptake of subconjunctivally injected C^{14} hydrocortisone. I. Time and major route of penetration in a normal eye. *Am. J. Ophthalmol.* 1964; **58**: 362–66.
10. McCartney HJ, Drysdale IO, Gornall AG and Basu PK. An autoradiographic study of the penetration of subconjunctivally injected hydrocortisone into the normal and inflamed rabbit eye. *Invest. Ophthalmol. Vis. Sci.* 1965; **4**: 297–302.
11. Lapalus P and Garraffo RG. Ocular pharmacokinetics. In: Hockwin O, Green KG and Rubin LF (eds) *Manual of Oculotoxicity Testing*, New York: Gustav Fischer Verlag 1992: 119–36.
12. Fraunfelder FT and Hanna C. Ophthalmic drug delivery systems. *Surv. Ophthalmol.* 1974; **18**: 292–98.
13. Fisher CA. Granuloma formation associated with subconjunctival injection of a corticosteroid in dogs. *J. Am. Vet. Med. Ass.* 1979; **174**: 1086–88.
14. Murphy CM, Lavach JD and Severin GA. Survey of conjunctival flora in dogs with clinical signs of external eye disease. *J. Am. Vet. Med. Ass.* 1978; **172**: 66–8.
15. Gerding PA, McLaughlin SA and Troop M. Pathogenic bacteria and

fungi associated with external ocular diseases in dogs: 131 cases (1981–1986). *J. Am. Vet. Med. Ass.* 1988; **193**: 242–44.

16. Petroutsos G, Savoldelli M and Pauliquen Y. The effect of gentamicin on the corneal endothelium. *Cornea* 1990; **9**: 62–5.

17. Moller I, Cook C, Peiffer RL, Nasisse MP and Harling DE. Indications for and complications of the pharmacological ablation of the ciliary body for the treatment of chronic glaucoma in the dog. *J. Am. Anim. Hosp. Ass.* 1986; **22**: 319–26.

18. Severin GA. *Severin's Veterinary Ophthalmology Notes,* 3rd edn. Fort Collins: Design Pointe Communications 1995: 88–9.

19. Noxon JO, Monroe WE and Chinn DR. Ketaconazole therapy in canine and feline cryptococcosis. *J. Am. Anim. Hosp. Ass.* 1986; **22**: 179.

20. Nasisse MP. Feline Ophthalmology. In: Gelatt KN (ed) *Veterinary Ophthalmology*, 2nd edn. Philadelphia: Lea & Febiger 1991: 539–41.

21. Weiss RC. Synergistic antiviral activities of acyclovir and recombinant human leukocyte (alpha) interferon on feline herpes virus replication. *Am. J. Vet. Res.* 1989: **50**: 1672–77.

22. Dow SW, Rosychuk RA, McChesney AE and Curtis CR. Effects of flunixin and flunixin plus prednisone on the gastrointestinal tracts of dogs. *Am. J. Vet. Res.* 1990; **51**: 1131–38.

23. Gwin RM, Gelatt KN, Gum GG and Peiffer RL. Effects of topical l-epinephrine and dipivalyl epinephrine on intraocular pressure and pupil size in the normotensive and glaucomatous beagle. *Am. J. Vet. Res.* 1978; **39**: 83–6.

24. Gumm GG, Larocca RD, Gelatt KN, Mead JP and Gelatt JK. The effect of topical timolol maleate on intraocular pressure in normal beagles and beagles with inherited glaucoma. *Prog. Vet. Comp. Ophthalmol.* 1991; **1**: 141–9.

25. Lui HK, Chiou GCY and Gorg LL. Ocular hypotensive effects of timolol in cat eyes. *Arch. Ophthalmol.* 1980; **98**: 1467–69.

26. Dugan SJ, Roberts SM and Severin GA. Systemic osmotherapy for ophthalmic disease in dogs and cats. *J. Am. Vet. Med. Ass.* 1989; **194**: 115–8.

27. Adams RE, Kirschner RJ and Leopold IH. Ocular hypotensive effect of intravenously administered mannitol. *Arch. Ophthalmol.* 1963; **69**: 55–8.

28. Scagliotti RH. Neuro-ophthalmology. In: Gelatt KN (ed). *Veterinary Ophthalmology*, 2nd edn. Philadelphia: Lea & Febiger 1991: 706–43.

29. Kaswan RL, Salisbury MA and Ward DA. Spontaneous canine keratoconjunctivitis: A model for human keratoconjunctivitis sicca – treatment with cyclosporine eye drops. *Arch. Ophthalmol.* 1989; **107**: 1210.

30. Jackson PA, Kaswan RL, Meredith RE and Barrett PM. Chronic superficial keratitis in dogs: A placebo controlled trial of topical cyclosporine treatment. *Prog. Vet. Comp. Ophthalmol.* 1991; **1**: 269–75.

31. Rubin LF and Aguirre GD. Clinical use of pilocarpine for keratoconjunctivitis in dogs and cats. *J. Am. Vet. Med. Ass.* 1969; **151**: 313.

32. Kleinfeld J and Ellis PP. Effects of topical anesthetics on growth of microorganisms. *Arch. Ophthalmol.* 1966; **76**: 712–15.

33. Roat ME, Romanowski E, Araullo-Cruz T and Gordon J. The antiviral effect of rose bengal and fluorescein. *Arch. Ophthalmol.* 1987; **105**: 1415–17.

34. da Silva Curiel JMA, Nasisse MP, Hook R, Wilson HH, Collins BK and Mandell CP. Topical fluorescein dye: effects on immunofluorescent antibody tests for feline herpesvirus keratoconjunctivitis. *Prog. Vet. Comp. Ophthalmol.* 1991; **1**: 99–104.

4

Abnormal Appearance

R. Gareth Jones and Peter Bedford

The conditions discussed in this chapter are those in which an alteration in the gross appearance of the eye is the primary presenting clinical feature. Other signs of disease may also be present and the reader should refer to other chapters in this book in cases where visual impairment, ocular pain, or ocular discharge are the most significant presenting signs. The first part of this chapter describes the normal appearance of the eye and adnexa (Figures 4.1 and 4.2) and abnormal appearance is discussed in the second part of the chapter.

NORMAL APPEARANCE

In the dog, in particular, selective breeding has resulted in a wide variation in the anatomical relationship between the skull, globe, and adnexa. Many of the resulting abnormalities are part of the breed

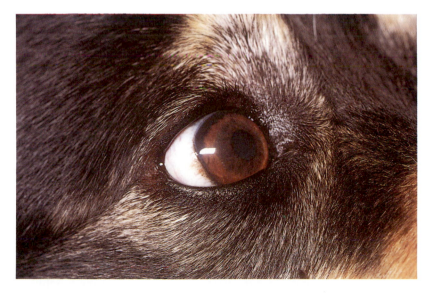

Figure 4.1 The normal appearance of the eye and adnexa in the dog. Right eye.

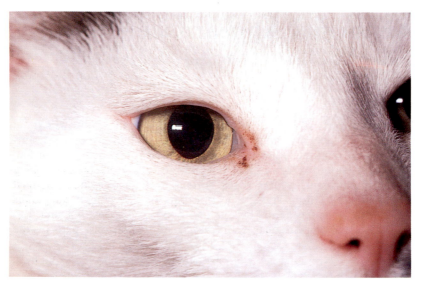

Figure 4.2   The normal appearance of the eye and adnexa in the cat. Right eye.

characteristics and are regarded as normal by the breeder. For example, the brachycephalic breeds are characterized by variable degrees of exophthalmos (an abnormally prominent globe) and lagophthalmos (a lack of complete eyelid closure) while lower lid ectropion to allow exposure of the third eyelid is a desired trait in the Bloodhound and St Bernard breeds. Age-related change also affects the ocular appearance, with atonic drooping of the palpebral fissure in the Cocker Spaniel or nuclear sclerosis of the lens in elderly dogs being the obvious examples to cite. The clinician should be aware of the influence of breed and age when conducting an ocular examination and must decide whether the presenting feature is simply an incidental finding, a conformational variation, or the indication of acquired disease which requires differential diagnosis and treatment.

The globe

The size of the globe, its position within the orbit, and the shape of the palpebral fissure all determine the overall external appearance of the eye. Accordingly, a relatively large globe in a shallow orbit results in the classical 'prominent eyed' appearance of the brachycephalic breeds, whereas a smaller globe set more deeply in the orbit is responsible for the typical appearance of the dolicocephalic dog.

Dogs with relatively small globes, deep orbits, and proportionally overlong palpebral fissures may exhibit deeply set eyes, protrusion of the third eyelid, and eyelid conformational anomalies.

The extraocular muscles primarily provide globe movement but also have some effect on the position of the globe within the orbit. Sympathetic innervation to orbital smooth muscle maintains the anterior position of the globe within the orbit, while the retractor bulbi muscles have an opposing effect.

The eyelids

The appearance and position of the eyelids are determined by a number of factors including the length of the palpebral fissure, support by the globe, and tension at the lateral canthus. However, cranium shape and mass of facial skin can alter this relationship, leading to conformational differences between the breeds. One example of an abnormality required by breed standards is the 'diamond eye' conformation in breeds like the St Bernard and the Bloodhound, where ectropion and third eyelid exposure can be responsible for chronic conjunctivitis.

In the normal animal, the eyelids should rest upon the ocular surface, their shape following the contour of the globe. They should move freely and fully across the corneal surface to complete the blink. Regular blinking is an essential feature of corneal physiology, being necessary to reform and spread the precorneal tear film effectively. The completion of blink and the rate of blinking can vary between species and breeds. The brachycephalic breeds blink less frequently and more incompletely than their dolicocephalic counterparts and often the central cornea is not adequately covered (lagophthalmos). This is due to the degree of exophthalmos present which, coupled with the relative insensitivity of the corneas of these breeds, predisposes to superficial keratitis and ulceration. Cats demonstrate both complete and incomplete blinking as a normal feature.

Tone within the orbicularis oculi and levator palpebrae superioris muscles, innervated by the facial nerve (VII) and the oculomotor nerve (III) respectively, also influence the appearance of the palpebral fissure. Senile atrophy of these muscles can result in a drooping of both the upper and lower eyelids, a condition seen most dramatically in the Cocker Spaniel breed. The resulting hooding effect of the upper eyelids may obscure vision and result in trichiasis/entropion, and the droop of the lower eyelid simply exposes the lower conjunctival sac.

The third eyelid

The third eyelid (membrana nictitans) lies against the anteriomedial aspect of the globe within the ventral intraorbital tissues and its position or degree of exposure is influenced by the globe size, the position of the globe within the orbit, the depth and contents of the orbit and the length of the palpebral fissure. In normality the third eyelid is positioned between the lower eyelid and the globe, protrusion being effected primarily by globe retraction. The normally pigmented leading edge of the membrana nictitans should be visible in the normal animal (Figure 4.3) but in some of the larger breeds and in dolicocephalic dogs it may be prominently displayed. It has the appearance of being more prominent when the leading edge lacks pigment, a normal feature in some animals (Figure 4.4). Loss of membrana pigment may be of clinical significance, but it also occurs as an age-related change. Third eyelid movement is passive in dogs, protrusion occurring when the globe is retracted, but in cats smooth muscle activity is responsible for some of the movement.

The conjunctiva/sclera

The conjunctiva is the transparent mucous membrane which lines the eyelids (palpebral conjunctiva) and covers the membrana nictitans (membrana conjunctiva) and the anterior sclera (bulbar conjunctiva). There is little variation between species and breeds. Pigmentation may be normal and is usually diffuse and irregular. It is important to appreciate the difference in normal appearance across the conjuncti-

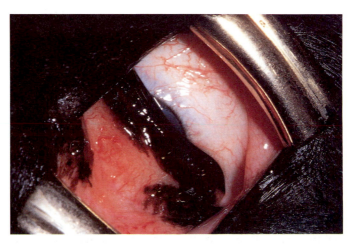

Figure 4.3   The normally pigmented leading edge of the membrana nictitans in a 2 year old German Shepherd dog. Left eye.

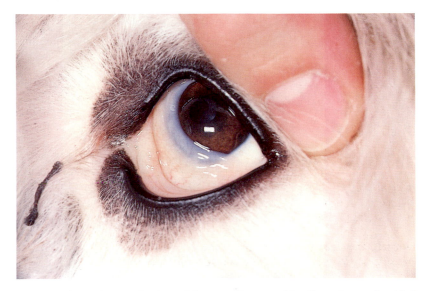

Figure 4.4 Left eye of a dog with a nonpigmented leading edge to the third eyelid.

val sac. The bulbar conjunctiva is loosely bound to the globe and it appears mainly white due to the color of the sclera beneath. Blood capillaries will be seen in the bulbar conjunctiva, sometimes imparting a salmon pink color. Elements of the underlying episcleral vasculature are not very prominent in the normal dog but are more readily seen in the cat. In contrast, the palpebral conjunctiva is firmly attached and its deep pink appearance is that of the underlying tarsal tissues (Figure 4.5), the conjunctiva within the fornix has a similar coloration but is loosely attached.

The cornea

The normal cornea is transparent and its anterior surface is optically smooth. The diameter varies from approximately 12.5–18mm in the dog and cat and the radius of curvature is approximately 8mm. The junction between the cornea and the sclera, the limbus is oblique, with the outer limbus overhanging the inner limbus maximally at the 12 and 6 o'clock positions.

Structurally, the cornea consists of a surface multilayered epithelium, a thicker middle layer, the stroma which is made up of collagen elements arranged in parallel lamellae, and an inner single layer of endothelium with its basement membrane, Descemet's membrane, separating it from the stroma. In order to allow it to be transparent, the cornea is avascular so nutrition must be supplied via the aqueous

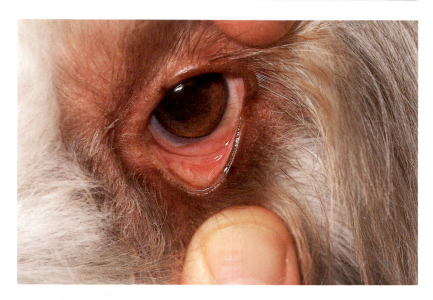

Figure 4.5   Comparison of the bulbar, palpebral, and membrana conjunctival surfaces. Left eye.

volume and to a lesser extent by the precorneal tear film and the limbal scleral and conjunctival vasculature. To remain transparent, the stroma is maintained in a relative state of dehydration and both the epithelium and endothelium are involved in this process. The epithelium presents a barrier to the tear film while an active endothelial pump mechanism regulates fluid exchange with the aqueous volume. In puppies and kittens, it is common for the cornea to appear cloudy immediately after the palpebral fissure first opens and until the endothelial 'pump' becomes fully functional.

Apart from maintaining ocular surface health, the precorneal tear film also has an important role in creating a smooth optical surface. This is demonstrated by the clean corneal reflection of an examining light on the normal eye. It is normal to see accumulated tear film debris at the medial canthus and where the canthus is deep and the lacrimal lake resultingly large, the amount of this accumulating 'sleep' may be considerable. This material should not be confused with the discharge of disease and it is commonly discussed by owners as a cause for concern.

The aqueous and the anterior chamber

The aqueous is a modified ultrafiltrate of blood and is normally transparent due to a low protein and cell content. It is produced by the ciliary processes, released into the posterior chamber and flows forwards between the iris and the lens through the pupil to fill the anterior chamber. There is little variation in the gross appearance of the normal anterior chamber between breeds but there are subtle variations in its depth which are difficult to appreciate during simple clinical examination.

The aqueous circulates thermodynamically within the anterior chamber and drains into the scleral vasculature through the 360° of the iridocorneal angle. In the domestic species, the angle extends into the ciliary body as the ciliary cleft. The entrance to the cleft is spanned by fibers of the pectinate ligament and its lumen contains the trabecular meshwork. The pectinate ligament may be visualized with the naked eye in the cat because of the considerable depth of the anterior chamber in this species, but this is not possible in the dog. In this species the use of a goniolens is required to examine the detail of the pectinate ligament and the entrance to the ciliary cleft. Between individuals, there is variation in both the amount of pigment in the scleral shelf and the physical structure of the pectinate ligament, both of which influence gonioscopic appearance. A wide pigmentary zone may render interpretation difficult on occasion but the pectinate ligament should always be visible in the normal animal.

Intraocular pressure (IOP) is maintained by homeostatic mechanisms resulting in an equilibrium between the rates of aqueous production and outflow. In young animals, the normal IOP is 15–30 mm Hg but this value can fall to below 10 mm Hg with age. However, the terrier breeds often have fluctuating high 'IOPs' that appear to be of no clinical significance.

The iris

Iris coloration is related to the density of coat and skin pigmentation and consequently demonstrates considerable variation between both species and breeds. Darker-coated breeds of dog will have a dark brown iris while in the subalbinotic breeds the iris is often blue (Figure 4.6). Yellow, green, and blue iris coloration can all be seen in cats (Figure 4.7). Iris pigment is located in the posterior pigment epithelium and the stroma; the outer or ciliary iridal zone tends to be darker than the inner pupillary zone. Heterochromia iridis describes a difference in color within the same iris or between the two irises of the same individual. Senile atrophy of the iris can result in a lace-like appearance demonstrable by transillumination. In addition, the pupillary light response may be sluggish or weak due to atrophy of the iris musculature.

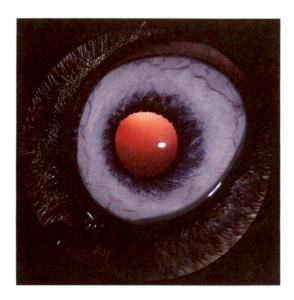

Figure 4.6   A blue iris demonstrating the difference in color density between the ciliary and pupillary zones in a 4 year old Siberian Husky. Left eye.

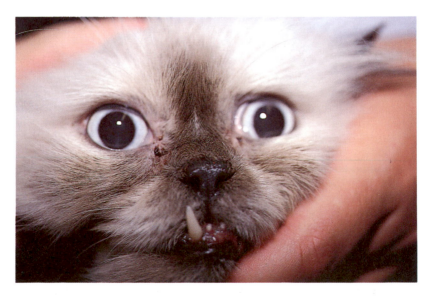

Figure 4.7   Blue iris color in a 2 year old cat.

The pupil

There is no variation in the appearance of the normal pupil between different breeds although shape does vary between species. The pupil is round in the dog and elliptical when constricted in the cat. There is often slight exposure of the darkly colored iris pigment epithelium at the pupil rim, an appearance described as ectropion uveae.

The pupil should dilate freely and maximally in the dark and constrict briskly and completely in bright light, this movement being the basis of assessment in the direct and consensual light reflexes. A ragged edge to the pupil can result from senile atrophy of the iris or the presence of posterior synechiae in which inflammation has produced adhesion between the lens capsule and the iris.

The lens

The position of the lens behind the iris means that only its axial portion is normally in view. Mydriatic drugs dilate the pupil and allow examination of the more equatorial parts of the lens. Their use is essential to allow a complete ophthalmic examination. The lens is a transparent structure and its presence between the vitreous body and the posterior surface of the iris is indicated by the forward bowing of the iris which rests on and slides over the anterior surface of the lens. Lens transparency is a function of the precise arrangement of the adult cortical lens fibers around the embryonic and fetal nucleus and, of course, the absence of blood vessels. Nutrition is by fluid exchange with the aqueous.

Suture lines mark the meeting points of lens fibers and in young animals opacities associated with the distal tips of the suture lines may be visible. These are termed 'false cataracts' as they disappear during the first few months of life. A normal aging feature of the lens is nuclear sclerosis in which refraction is altered as the central nuclear material becomes progressively more compressed by continuous secondary lens fiber formation. Distant direct ophthalmoscopy should readily differentiate this apparent opacity from a true cataract as there is no real opacity to interfere with the tapetal reflection.

The posterior segment

The fundus is divided into tapetal and non-tapetal areas. The non-tapetal area occupies the major proportion of the fundus and this area is usually darkly colored due to pigment within the retinal pigment epithelium and the underlying choroid. Retinal pigment epithelium which overlies the reflective brightly-colored tapetum is non-pigmented. Tapetal color varies, but most commonly is yellow, orange, green, or blue (Figure 4.8). The tapetum may be small or completely absent, particularly in the toy breeds and a 'red' reflex is normal in

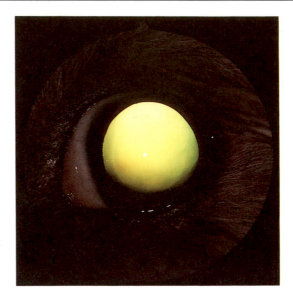

Figure 4.8   A yellow-green tapetal reflex in a 4-year-old crossbred dog.

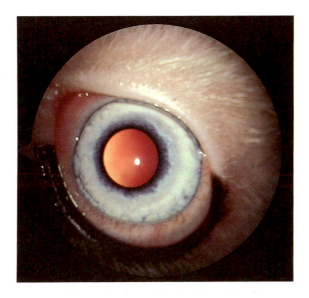

Figure 4.9   The red tapetal reflex due to subalbinism in a 2-year-old Old English Sheepdog.

subalbinotic breeds which may lack a tapetum in addition to reduced or absent retinal pigment epithelium and choroidal pigment (Figure 4.9). Inflammatory product within the vitreous or retina will reduce the intensity of the tapetal reflex and where the retina is degenerate or totally detached the reflectivity will be increased. In the presence of extensive retinal degeneration there will be a loss of the pupillary light reflex which enhances the appearance of the increased reflection from the affected eye.

ABNORMAL APPEARANCE

The eye should never be examined in isolation and the examination itself should be systematic. The most significant changes in appearance are listed alphabetically in Table 4.1. Each clinical sign listed in Table 4.1 will be discussed in terms of investigation, diagnosis, and treatment.

The globe

Prominence of the globe

Exophthalmos is the protrusion of a normal-sized globe from its usual position (Figure 4.10). The history should establish whether the condition is acute or chronic and whether it appeared spontaneously or was associated with known trauma. The presence of pain can be an important indication that inflammatory disease is the cause. During the examination it will be seen that the palpebral fissure is noticeably wider than normal and complete eyelid closure may not be possible. A comparison of the position of each globe, particularly from above, is usually sufficient to determine the degree of displacement. Prominence of the membrana nictitans and resistance to retropulsion will differentiate exophthalmos from buphthalmos.

Examination of the oral cavity caudal to the last upper molar tooth may reveal extension of a retrobulbar tumor, the draining sinus of a retrobulbar abscess, or distension due to zygomatic mucocele formation.

Radiography may only reveal non-specific soft tissue swelling although an occlusal view of the nasal cavity is important in the investigation of nasal tumors which can erode through the orbital wall to influence the position of the globe. Periosteal changes will be seen in craniomandibular osteopathy. Ultrasound examination will confirm the presence of a retrobulbar mass and may give some indication of the tissue type involved according to its ultrasonographic appearance[1]. In addition, imaging techniques such as MRI (magnetic resonance imaging) can be valuable. Fine needle

Table 4.1   Abnormal appearance

Globe

Prominence (exophthalmos):	arteriovenous fistula (rare), orbital fracture, retrobulbar space-occupying lesion (e.g. masticatory myositis, neoplasia, retrobulbar abscess/cellulitis, zygomatic mucocele) temporomandibular osteopathy, traumatic proptosis.
Recession (enophthalmos):	Horner's syndrome, loss of retrobulbar fat (debility, senility), orbital fracture, severe ocular pain, temporal muscle atrophy.
Small globe:	globe rupture, microphthalmos, phthisis bulbi.
Enlarged globe:	glaucoma, neoplasia.

Eyelids

Alopecia:	bacterial pyoderma, immune mediated disease, mycoses, nutritional disease, parasitic infestation, seborrhoea.
Swellings/masses:	abscess, allergy, epibulbar dermoid, neoplasia, ophthalmia neonatorum, trauma.
Shape of palpebral fissure:	coloboma, ectropion, entropion, combined ectropion/entropion (diamond eye), laceration.

Membrana Nictitans

Prominence:	anterior segment pain, dysautonomia, Horner's syndrome, retrobulbar lesion, sedation, Haws syndrome, symblepharon, systemic disease (e.g. tetanus).
Distortion:	prolapse of the nictitans gland, scrolling of the cartilage.
Masses:	lymphoid follicles, neoplasia, plasma cell infiltration.

Conjunctiva/sclera

Redness:	conjunctivitis (superficial), ciliary flush/episcleral congestion (deep), episcleritis (deep), subconjunctival hemorrhage.
Swelling:	allergy, conjunctivitis, diffuse neoplasia.
Masses:	cyst, neoplasia, nodular episcleritis.

Cornea

Opacity:	edema (white/blue), pigmentation (black), scarring (blue/gray), vascularization (red).
Masses:	dermoid, granulation tissue, infiltrative neoplasms.
Vascularization:	corneal infiltration and degeneration, eosinophilic keratitis, healing ulcer, herpes keratitis, immune mediated disease, sequestrum, superficial and deep keratitis, trauma.
Infiltration:	calcareous degeneration, corneal 'melting' ulcer, lipidosis, (dystrophy, degeneration, and infiltration), neoplasia.

Change in contour: bullous keratopathy, corneal abscess, corneal laceration, descemetocele, inclusion cyst, iris prolapse.

Loss of tissue: laceration, ulceration.

Anterior chamber

Turbidity: lipid-laden aqueous, uveitis (flare/hypopyon, keratitic precipitates, hyphema).

Masses: foreign body, lens luxation, neoplasia, uveal cyst.

Hyphema: blood dyscrasias, chronic glaucoma, congenital lesions, hypertension, neoplasia, retinal detachment, trauma, uveitis.

Iris

Discoloration: chronic uveitis (pigmentation), portosystemic shunt (rare), rubeosis iridis (vascularization).

Masses: neoplasia, uveal cysts.

'Strands': persistent pupillary membrane, synechiae.

Pupil

Dilated: coloboma, dysautonomia, fear, glaucoma, iris atrophy, oculomotor nerve lesion, optic neuropathy, pharmacological agents, retinopathy.

Constricted: Horner's syndrome, pharmacological agents, uveitis.

Distorted: coloboma, iridodonesis, synechiae.

Lens

Opacification: cataract, uveitis (anterior capsular pigment), nuclear sclerosis, persistent hyperplastic primary vitreous (hemorrhage).

Position: luxation, subluxation.

Posterior segment

Leukocoria (white pupil): cataract, intraocular foreign body, neoplasia, persistent hyperplastic primary vitreous, retinal detachment, vitreous abscess.

Increased reflectivity (plus dilated pupil): retinal degeneration, retinal detachment with disinsertion.

Decreased reflectivity: posterior uveitis (vitreous haze), bullous retinal detachment.

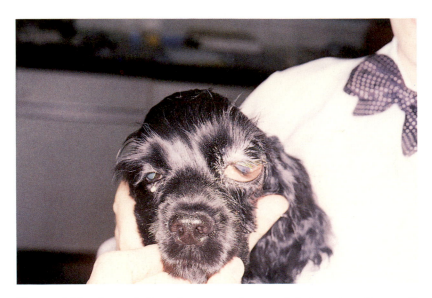

Figure 4.10 A retrobulbar abscess causing exophthalmos in a 6-year-old American Cocker Spaniel.

aspiration biopsy may allow a cytological diagnosis while exploratory orbitotomy may be necessary to confirm the exact nature and extent of the orbital pathology [2].

The prognosis for most orbital tumors is poor. It is uncommon for a tumor to be removable via an orbitotomy without enucleation. Usually orbital exenteration (removal of globe and orbital contents) is required and in many patients even this is not curative. Lateral orbitotomy enables extirpation of the zygomatic salivary gland when mucocoele formation is the cause of the exophthalmos.

Traumatic proptosis of the globe

Traumatic proptosis in which there is prolapse of the globe through the palpebral fissure is usually associated with known trauma (Figure 4.11). Minor trauma such as scruffing or dog fights may result in proptosis in the brachycephalic breeds, but proptosis in the dolicocephalic breeds requires considerable trauma. Various criteria including the absence of the pupillary light reflex and the degree of intraocular damage are used to determine the prognosis for vision; often the eye is blind due to the accompanying optic neuropathy [3]. Following prolapse the cornea must be kept moist whilst any life-threatening injuries are dealt with. Once the animal can be safely anesthetized the globe is replaced; a lateral canthotomy to enlarge the palpebral fissure will facilitate the procedure. A temporary tarsorrhaphy is then performed to maintain the

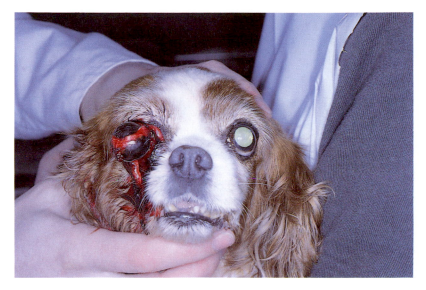

Figure 4.11 Traumatic proptosis of the right eye in a 5 year old Cavalier King Charles Spaniel. Complete avulsion of the optic nerve has occurred.

globe *in situ*. The sutures are not removed until the orbital swelling subsides and lid movement is noted. Lateral (divergent) strabismus is a common sequel due to oculomotor nerve damage or avulsion of the medial rectus muscle (Figure 4.12). If corneoscleral rupture, lens luxation, optic nerve avulsion, or rupture of all the extraocular muscles has occurred then enucleation will prove necessary.

Globe enlargement

Buphthalmos is an acquired enlargement of the globe due to glaucoma. It should be differentiated from exophthalmos, although this is usually straightforward. The cardinal signs of glaucoma are a dilated non-responsive pupil, episcleral congestion, corneal edema, and elevated intraocular pressure. Degenerative corneal changes may accompany chronic glaucoma, and tears in Descemet's membrane (Haab's striae) are a sure indication of increased globe size. The presence of optic nerve atrophy and retinal degeneration render the prognosis for vision poor. For sighted eyes, the control of intraocular pressure may be attempted as discussed in Chapter 6. For permanently blind eyes, a number of methods of ciliary body destruction are available to reduce the IOP permanently. These include cyclocryotherapy, photocoagulation, and pharmacological ablation using intracameral gentamicin. Evisceration and implantation of silicone prostheses or enucleation offer alternative approaches [4]. In every instance the etiology of the

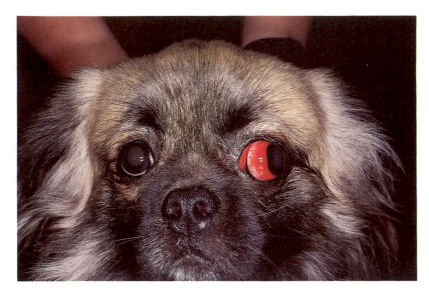

Figure 4.12   Acquired strabismus following traumatic proptosis in a 3 year old Tibetan Spaniel. Rupture of the medial rectus muscle has occurred. Left eye.

glaucoma should be established and the possibility of the presence of an intraocular tumor resulting in secondary glaucoma ruled out.

Strabismus

Strabismus is a deviation in the position of the globe. It can be due to a congenital anomaly, a neurological lesion, or abnormality of the extraocular muscles. Congenital esotropia (bilateral medial strabismus) is seen in Siamese cats. Acquired strabismus may result from traumatic proptosis or retrobulbar lesions (Figure 4.12). Lesions of the III, IV, or VI cranial nerves will produce a specific deviation. Treatment is not usually necessary.

Nystagmus

Nystagmus is an involuntary oscillatory movement of the eyes. The movement is made up of repeated slow and fast phases. During the slow phase the eyes move away from the primary gaze position (looking straight ahead), this is followed by the fast phase which recenters the eyes. Normal nystagmus can be induced as a response to movement of the head (acceleration or deceleration), for example, in the oculocephalic reflex. Abnormal nystagmus is associated with central or peripheral vestibular disease and in some cases only occurs when the animal's head is moved in to a particular position (positional nystagmus) or it may be present without needing to interfere with the head position (spontaneous nystagmus). Animals with congenital multiocular anomalies (e.g. microphthalmos, persistent pupillary membranes, and cataracts), or conditions resulting in a very early-onset of blindness often show abnormal eye movements of an oscillatory or wandering nature described as a searching nystagmus. Cerebellar disease can also result in a form of nystagmus.

Recession of the globe

Enophthalmos describes the recession of a normal-sized globe into the orbit. There is associated prominence of the third eyelid and possible deviation in the shape of the palpebral fissure. Retraction of the globe as a result of pain is a common cause. If enophthalmos follows trauma, the clinician should check to see if the globe has been perforated (the eye will be hypotensive) or if there are periorbital fractures (by palpation or radiography). Enophthalmos may also result from loss of retrobulbar fat in cachexic states, the presence of retrobulbar scar tissue or chronic, postmyositic masticatory muscle wasting. The history and clinical signs should make the diagnosis obvious and treatment is addressed to the cause.

Horner's syndrome is a common cause of enophthalmos, the cardinal signs being ptosis, miosis, enophthalmos, and third eyelid protrusion (Figure 4.13). The signs are specific and an attempt should

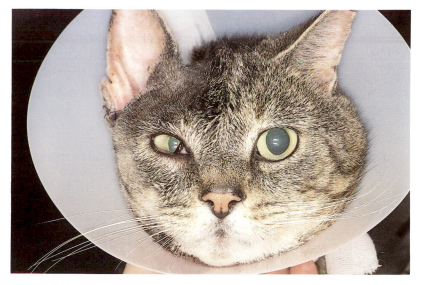

Figure 4.13 Third order Horner's syndrome following bulla osteotomy in a 4 year old Domestic Short-Haired (DSH) cat. The signs of ptosis, miosis, enophthalmos, and membrana nictitans protrusion are present in the right eye.

be made to localize the lesion [5]. Pharmacological testing with phenylephrine can give an indication as to whether the lesion is central (first order), preganglionic (second order), or postganglionic (third order). Pupillary dilation and third eyelid retraction following topical application of 10% phenylephrine occurs within 20 min with third order Horner's syndrome, whilst it takes 45 min with second order lesions and considerably longer with third order lesions. Common causes of Horner's syndrome include middle ear disease, iatrogenic damage resulting from middle ear surgery, puncture wounds to the neck, and less commonly polyneuropathies, tumors, and brachial plexus avulsions. In many instances the etiology remains obscure and in the Golden Retriever in the UK there appears to be a relatively high incidence of an idiopathic Horner's syndrome.

An abnormally small globe

The presence of a congenitally small globe is termed microphthalmos. Often this condition is seen as part of a multiocular anomaly together with nystagmus, persistence of pupillary membrane, cataract, and in some instances retinal dysplasia (see p. 106). There is a breed predisposition in the dog but this condition will be seen randomly throughout the animal world. The cataract is usually nonprogressive and the eyes are often visual.

Penetrating trauma may lead to a collapse of the globe. Complete ocular examination should be diagnostic and repair can be successful. Phthisis bulbi denotes an irreversibly damaged and shrunken eye. It is a common sequel to severe injury, chronic uveitis, or glaucoma. Such eyes are blind and enucleation is indicated if the eye becomes a persistent focus of discomfort. There is a recorded incidence of sarcoma development in phthisical feline globes.

The eyelids

Congenital/neonatal eyelid conditions

A coloboma is a congenital absence of tissue at any depth within the eye or its adnexa. Any part of the eyelid may be involved (Figure 4.14), but in the cat such lesions usually involve the lateral part of the upper eyelid. The absence of eyelid margin is obvious and hair bearing skin will be seen fused to the bulbar conjunctiva adjacent to the cornea, obliterating most of the dorsal conjunctival fornix. Eyelid closure is not complete and exposure keratitis results. Blepharoplastic techniques are necessary for the correction of the deformity, but success in producing an adequate blink depends on the amount of normal eyelid present.

Epibulbar dermoid is a congenital mass of hair-bearing skin situated in an abnormal location. It may involve the eyelid, the

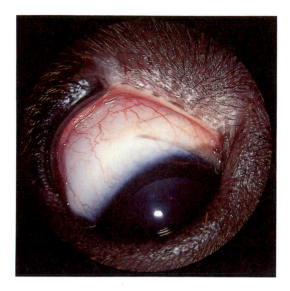

Figure 4.14 A coloboma involving the medial aspect of the upper eyelid in a 4 month old terrier cross. Right eye.

conjunctiva, the cornea, or all three. Treatment is by resection, keratectomy, or blepharoplastic repair depending on the location.

Fusion of the eyelids or ankyloblepharon is normal in kittens and puppies up to 10–14 days of age, but on occasion it may persist beyond this time necessitating surgical separation of the fused lids. Ophthalmia neonatorum describes the development of a purulent conjunctivitis prior to eyelid opening which results in a swelling of the palpebral area. Early intervention is required to avoid damage to the cornea or even loss of the eye. The accumulated pus is drained by opening the lids and irrigating the conjunctival sac. Broad spectrum topical antibiotics are then applied to control bacterial infection and keep the ocular surface moist until tear production is established.

Abnormality of eyelid conformation is common and often breed related. An inward rolling of the eyelid is called entropion while an eversion is termed ectropion. In entropion the friction caused by the movement of the hair bearing skin in blinking can result in superficial keratitis and corneal ulceration. Surgical intervention is required to correct the eyelid deformity (suitable procedures are described on p. 171–173). Ectropion leads to chronic exposure of the ventral conjunctival sac and may lead to permanent conjunctival changes. Several techniques are available for the correction of ectropion when this proves to be necessary but complete correction can be difficult; the majority of cases are readily controlled with daily irrigation with sterile saline and periodic use of lubricant ointments [6].

Acquired eyelid lesions

Traumatic lacerations of the eyelids require accurate surgical repair using minimal debridement and the treatment of any secondary infection.

Blepharitis has a number of possible causes including bacterial pyoderma, immune-mediated disease, mycotic infection, parasitic infestation, and seborrhoea [7]. Specific diagnosis depends on skin scrapings and bacteriological culture. Treatment is by systemic antibiotics, antifungals, corticosteroids, and antiparasitic drugs where indicated. The initial blepharitis is often exacerbated by self trauma and measures should be taken to control this as part of the management of the condition.

Swellings or masses of the eyelids may be due to abscess formation (styes), allergy, epibulbar dermoid, neoplasia, ophthalmia neonatorum, and trauma (Figure 4.15). Styes result from abscesses of the perifollicular glands of the cilia and require treatment with systemic antibiotics, hot compresses, and possibly surgical drainage. Retention and the resulting inspissation of meibomian lipid creates a pocket of hardened secretion surrounded by an inflammatory reaction known as a chalazion. Removal of the inspissated material via an incision through the overlying conjunctiva is required.

Eyelid tumors in the dog are usually benign, the commonest being sebaceous adenomas. Benign tumors involving up to approximately

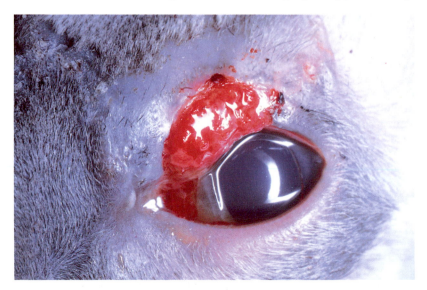

Figure 4.15   A mast cell tumor involving the upper eyelid in a 10-year-old Siamese cat. Left eye.

one-third the length of an eyelid with normal conformation can be treated successfully by wedge resection and direct two-layer closure. Removal of larger tumors may require more elaborate reconstructive procedures. Eyelid tumors in cats are more commonly malignant and include squamous cell carcinoma, basal cell carcinoma, and fibrosarcoma. The invasive malignancies require wide margin excision or a more aggressive treatment such as cryotherapy.

Facial paralysis results in a loss of the palpebral reflex and if the parasympathetic supply to the lacrimal and nictitans glands which passes in the initial portion of the facial nerve is affected there may also be reduced tear production. Unilateral facial nerve paralysis may be idiopathic or associated with erosive middle ear disease such as severe infection or tumor. Bilateral lesions may be idiopathic although systemic conditions, such as hypothyroidism, which may be associated with neuropathies should be ruled out. Severe corneal changes result if there is an accompanying lack of tear production or if, when the animal attempts to blink, retraction of the globe with resultant sweeping of the third eyelid across the cornea cannot adequately spread the tear film. Brachycephalic dogs with their prominent globes, shallow orbits, and limited passive movement of the third eyelid are likely to develop exposure keratopathy as a result of facial paralysis. Topical tear replacements should be applied frequently until the normal eyelid movement is restored.

The third eyelid

Prominence of the third eyelid

Prominence of the third eyelid is most commonly caused by anterior segment pain and treatment is thus directed towards the cause (see Chapter 6). Others causes of protrusion include sedation, dehydration, 'Haws' syndrome (associated with viral diarrhea), Horner's syndrome (see above), retrobulbar lesions, symblepharon, dysautonomia, and systemic disease (e.g. tetanus).

Scrolling of the third eyelid

The shape of the third eyelid may be distorted by a scrolling of its cartilage, the free margin of the membrana usually rolling outwards (Figure 4.16). The covering conjunctiva can become inflamed and the shape of the palpebral fissure may be distorted. There may be epiphora due to an inability to pool tears in the medial lacrimal lake and to complete the blink. Correction requires resection of the distorted portion of the cartilage, usually leaving the crossbar of this T-shaped structure intact by removing a section of the stem just below the crossbar.

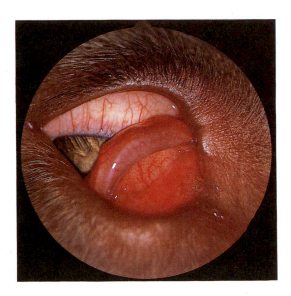

Figure 4.16   Scrolling of the membrana cartilage in a 6-month-old Weimaraner. Right eye.

Prolapse of the nictitans gland

The base of the membrana cartilage is enveloped by the nictitans gland which produces a proportion of the precorneal tear film. Occasionally in dogs with a loose palpebral fissure, the brachycephalic breeds, other breeds with genetic predisposition (beagles, American cockers, English bulldogs), and rarely in cats, the nictitans gland can prolapse upwards between the posterior surface of the membrana and the cornea to appear at the medial canthus (Figure 4.17). Here it presents as a smooth-surfaced, ellipsoidal mass which may become congested and inflamed. There is often an accompanying epiphora due to the functional loss of the medial lacrimal lake. Diagnosis is straightforward and treatment requires the surgical repositioning of the gland either by anchoring it to the ventromedial orbital rim (Figure 4.18) [8] or by performing a 'pocketing' procedure [9]. Gland excision should be avoided as this may adversely influence the nature of the precorneal tear film.

Other third eyelid conditions

Other conditions altering the appearance of the third eyelid include lymphoid follicles, plasmacytic conjunctivitis, and neoplasia. It is normal for the bulbar surface of the third eyelid to have a roughened appearance due to conjunctival lymphoid tissue overlying the nicti-

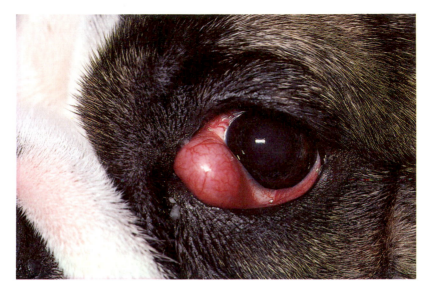

Figure 4.17 Prolapse of the nictitans gland in a 4-month-old Bulldog. Left eye.

tans gland. Proliferation of lymphoid follicles tends to occur in young dogs, apparently as a non-specific response and is often accompanied by mild irritation and a mucoid discharge. Debridement of excessive lymphoid follicles has been suggested. Plasmacytic conjunctivitis is commonest in German Shepherd dogs and may accompany chronic superficial keratitis. The exposed portion of the third eyelid is affected and may be thickened, have an irregular border and be depigmented. There may be a seromucoid discharge. Topical cyclosporine controls this immune-mediated condition. Tumors involving the nictitating membrane include squamous cell carcinoma, fibrosarcoma, adenomas or adenocarcinomas, and hemangiomas or hemangiosarcomas.

The conjunctiva/sclera

In disease the conjunctival surfaces and superficial scleral tissues are subjected to visible vascular change and swelling due to generalized inflammation or localized mass formation. Conjunctivitis is inflammation of the conjunctiva and may be caused by allergy, eyelid lesions, foreign bodies, immune-mediated disease, infections, irritants, precorneal tear film deficiency, and trauma (see Chapter 7). The cardinal sign of conjunctivitis is a red, discharging eye which itches rather than hurts. Conjunctival tissues may become edematous and considerable swelling is possible; on occasion, and particularly in cats, this chemosis may mask the cornea. However, conjunctivitis is a

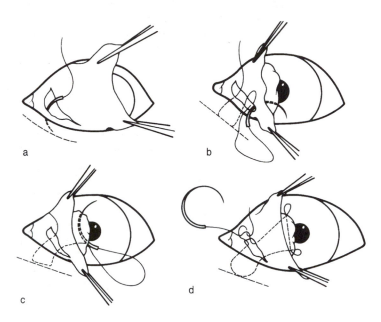

Figure 4.18   Diagram showing correction of prolapse of the nictitans gland by suturing to the orbital rim. (a) Allis tissue forceps are gently applied to the periphery of the free margin of the third eyelid and it is pulled across the eye. An incision is made in the medioventral conjunctival fornix (at the base of the third eyelid) using scissors. Blunt dissection allows access to the periosteum of the medioventral orbital rim. A firm bite of periosteum along the orbital rim is taken using 3/0 'PDS' (Ethicon), or monofilament nylon, suture with a swaged on needle introduced through the previously made incision. It can be difficult to obtain a bite of periosteum and bring the needle out through the incision, because access to the areas is limited. (b) The needle is then passed through the original incision dorsally towards the prolapsed gland so as to emerge from the glands at its most prominent point of prolapse. (c) With the third eyelid everted, the needle is passed back through the exit hole in the gland to take a horizontal bite from the most prominent part of the gland. (d) Finally the needle is passed back through the last exit hole to emerge through the original incision in the conjunctival fornix, thus encircling a large portion of the glands. The suture ends are tied. This creates a suture loop through the gland which anchors it to the periosteum of the orbital rim preventing it from re-prolapsing. The conjunctival incision can now be repaired using 6/0 'vicryl' (Ethicon) or it may be left unsutured. Postoperatively topical antibiotic cover is given.

Redrawn with permission from Petersen-Jones SM. Conditions of the eyelid and nictitating membrane. In: Petersen-Jones SM & Crispin SM (eds) *Manual of Small Animal Ophthalmology*, Cheltenham: British Small Animal Veterinary Association Publications 1993: 65–90.

common misdiagnosis and complete ophthalmic examination is indicated in every case, giving due consideration to other causes of the 'red eye'. The differential diagnoses for the 'red eye' are conjunctivitis, uveitis, glaucoma, episcleritis, and neoplasia [10]. The dorsal bulbar surface of the eye should be examined closely and the depth and degree of involvement of the conjunctival and episcleral vasculature determined (Figure 4.19). The episcleral vessels run at 90° to the limbus and congestion usually indicates the presence of intraocular disease such as uveitis or glaucoma. Congestion of the conjunctival vessels may also be present and careful examination is necessary to identify the true nature of the underlying lesion. Inflammation of the episclera may be localized (nodular episcleritis) or more generalized and may also involve the cornea. The management of uveitis and glaucoma are considered in Chapter 6. Episcleritis is usually treated with corticosteroids and if necessary immunosupressive drugs such as azathioprine.

An uncommon disease presumed to be an immunorelated process is seen in Doberman Pinschers and Golden Retrievers. The ocular lesions appear as a bilateral yellow-green membrane lining any or all of the conjunctival surfaces; stripping the ulcer away leaves a roughened and ulcerated epithelial surface. Exfoliative cytology reveals inflammatory cells with a prominent eosinophilic component; the membrane itself is composed of epithelial cells and a proteinaceous exudate. Variable associated systemic signs include proteinuria and ulcerative lesions of the skin and other mucus membranes; notably the oral cavity. This enigmatic condition can be

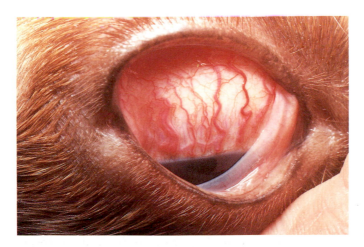

Figure 4.19 Acute 'closed angle' glaucoma demonstrating episcleral congestion in a 4-year-old Welsh Springer Spaniel. Right eye.

controlled in most cases with topical corticosteroids as well as systemic corticosteroids and/or azothioprine.

Conjunctival adhesions (symblepharon) may result from severe conjunctivitis. In cats the commonest cause is feline herpesvirus infection in kittens. The inflamed conjunctiva may adhere to itself, possibly obliterating the conjunctival fornices and interfering with tear drainage. Third eyelid movement may be reduced by adhesions, or the third eyelid may even be fixed partly across the eye. Adhesions to the cornea also occur, with scarred conjunctiva being drawn onto the corneal surface. Apart from the change in appearance of the affected eye there will often be a tear overflow and sometimes a mucoid to mucopurulent discharge and occasionally recurrent inflammation. Surgery to breakdown the adhesions is best reserved for the more severely affected animals (e.g. those with visual impairment) because adhesions will often reform after surgery. This tendency can be reduced by the postoperative application of a therapeutic contact lens.

The most common congenital mass is the dermoid. Acquired masses include neoplasia (squamous cell carcinoma, limbal melanoma), conjunctival cysts, and nodular episcleritis.

The cornea

Loss of transparency is readily diagnosed and may result from fluid accumulation, pigmentation, vascularization, symblepharon, endothelial deposits, or stromal lipid deposition.

Corneal edema

Corneal edema occurs if there is a break in the anatomical or functional integrity of the corneal epithelium or endothelium. It is commonly seen in corneal ulceration in which the loss of epithelium allows the adjacent stroma to soak up fluid from the tear film (Figure 4.20). Canine adenovirus I infection (or historical use of a live CAV1 vaccine) can result in corneal edema due to immune-complex deposition affecting corneal endothelial cells. The edema may be transient and resolve completely if the concurrent uveitis is treated, but it can lead to permanent opacity. Corneal endothelial degeneration may also result from intraocular disease such as anterior uveitis or glaucoma, drug toxicity (e.g. tocainide hydrochloride), or inherited endothelial dystrophy. The latter condition occurs in Boston Terriers, English Springer Spaniels, Chihuahuas, Dachshunds, miniature Poodles, and occasionally other breeds, usually affecting middle-aged animals. It has also been observed in young cats. The resulting progressive edema eventually involves the whole cornea. In severely affected patients, fluid-filled epithelial bullae may

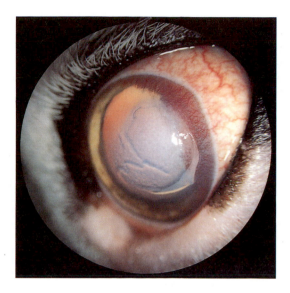

Figure 4.20 Ulcerative keratitis and corneal edema due to epithelial dystrophy in a 4-year-old Boxer. Left eye.

form and rupture to leave a superficial ulcer. In the cat an idiopathic usually bilateral focal edema with large bullae has been described. Differential diagnosis of corneal edema necessitates a complete ophthalmic examination which includes tonometry and, where possible, gonioscopy.

Treatment of corneal edema is aimed at the specific cause. With resolution of the ulcer or the keratitis the corneal opacity will clear, although scarring may result in some persistent opacity. Topical hyperosmotics such as sodium chloride ointment may temporarily reduce the degree of edema in patients with endothelial dystrophy, but as endothelial cells do not repair and are not replaced, the prognosis is poor. Penetrating keratoplasty may be the only hope of obtaining a clearer cornea in these patients. Third eyelid flaps are beneficial in cats with acute bullous keratopathy.

Corneal pigmentation

Corneal pigmentation may be seen in chronic keratitis, particularly in the brachycephalic breeds where lagophthalmos or trichiasis such as corneal contact with nasal folds may be the predisposing factors. In *keratitis pigmentosa* there is a chronic, superficial deposition of melanin associated with a low-grade vascularization. The process starts in early life with pigment appearing at the medial limbus and

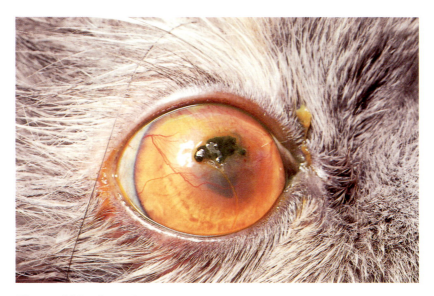

Figure 4.21   Corneal sequestrum in a 4 year old Burmese cat. Right eye.

with time there is a gradual spread of pigment deposition across the cornea towards the lateral limbus.

Corneal sequestrum is a disease peculiar to cats, with characteristic lesions ranging from brown discoloration of the cornea to formation of a dense black plaque of variable size consisting of necrotic corneal stroma (Figure 4.21). The condition may be unilateral or bilateral and often the dense plaques eventually slough. The etiopathogenesis remains open to speculation but many cases are associated with ulcerative keratitis [11] and in others feline herpesvirus may play a role. Corneal sequestra which cause discomfort are removed by keratectomy and if the resulting corneal defect is deep a conjunctival pedicle flap is applied. The conjunctival flap may help to prevent a recurrence of the lesion.

Limbal melanomas may infiltrate the cornea as well as the sclera and appear as raised black lesions which tend to be slow growing. They must be differentiated from intraocular melanomas eroding through the ocular coats. Treatment by excision with or without a graft, laser, or cryosurgery is required for the progressive lesions.

Staphylomas, which are the protrusion of uveal tissue through a corneal or scleral defect initially may appear black or, occasionally, brown due to a covering of fibrin. They may be congenital, traumatic, or secondary to chronic glaucoma.

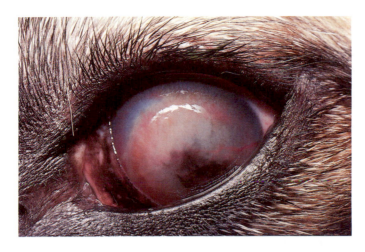

Figure 4.22 Chronic superficial keratitis in an 8 year old German Shepherd dog. The marked corneal vascularization and pigmentation indicate chronicity. Left eye.

Corneal vascularization

Corneal vascularization is a common pathological reaction to a number of different insults. These include precorneal tear film deficiency, eyelid abnormalities, trauma, infections, chemical irritants, immune-mediated disease, and diseases primarily involving adjacent structures; for example, episcleritis, scleritis, anterior uveitis, and glaucoma. It is useful when investigating the cause of the inflammation to differentiate between superficial and deep corneal vascularization. Deeper vessels tend to branch less, are darker in color and their origins from scleral vessels are obscured by the scleral overhang at the limbus, whereas superficial vessels can be seen crossing the limbus after arising from conjunctival vessels.

The possibility of concurrent corneal ulceration should be considered when keratitis is present and staining with fluorescein forms part of the investigation.

Chronic superficial keratitis (CSK) in the dog, often referred to as pannus, is an immune-mediated condition characterized by progressive, superficial, densely vascularized corneal inflammatory lesions [12]. CSK occurs bilaterally, with the lesions first developing in the ventrolateral quadrant of the cornea. Initially there is a corneal inflammatory cell infiltrate accompanied by vascularization, which progresses at a variable rate to produce thick superficial corneal granulation tissue. The lesion may eventually involve the majority of the cornea and result in severe visual impairment. There is a variable degree of pigmentation of the lesions and in long-standing cases scar tissue is present (Figure 4.22). Exposure to ultraviolet light is a predisposing factor for CSK. Treatment consists of topical cyclosporine or corticosteroids. Subconjunctival depocorticosteroids are useful in more severe cases. Owners should be made aware of the likelihood of exacerbation and the need for long-term treatment. When the degree of irreversible corneal change is extensive enough to reduce vision, a superficial keratectomy may be required or, if available, applications of beta-radiation. Following keratectomy the cornea often revascularizes surprisingly rapidly and to control this cyclosporine and possibly even corticosteroid treatment should be continued during the healing phase.

Eosinophilic keratitis, a condition unique to the cat, results in a progressive, superficial, corneal inflammatory lesion with a surface deposit of a white 'cottage cheese-like' material. Any part of the cornea may be involved as may the adjacent conjunctiva; the condition may be unilateral or bilateral. Eosinophilic keratitis is controlled by topical corticosteroids or cyclosporine. Unlike many cases of CSK the lesions can resolve completely with treatment, although like CSK they may recur.

Symblepharon is another cause of corneal opacity in which a vascularized whitish/grey membrane is adherent to the corneal surface and is discussed in depth above with conditions causing abnormal appearance of the conjunctiva.

Corneal denervation (lesions of ophthalmic branch of trigeminal V) results in a reduced blink reflex, which combined with loss of the trophic effect that normal sensory innervation has on corneal epithelium leads to neurotrophic keratitis. This is characterized by superficial vascularization and often serious ulceration affecting the cornea within the palpebral fissure.

Non-specific keratitis can be treated using corticosteroids, provided there is no evidence of corneal ulceration. It should be remembered that vascularization will occur as a normal component of stromal healing and should not be suppressed inappropriately.

Corneal lipid and calcium deposition

The deposition of lipid in the stroma is described as corneal lipidosis. It may be due to dystrophic or degenerative conditions of the cornea or it may be associated with several hyperlipidemic disease processes [13]. Crystalline stromal dystrophy is characterized by central, subepithelial oval or circular opacities, often with a 'ground glass' appearance, in an otherwise normal cornea (Figure 4.23). It is typically bilateral although may initially be unilateral. Lesions may slowly alter in size but generally have no effect on vision and require no treatment. A number of breeds of dog are affected and in some it has been shown to be familial. Siberian Huskys suffer from a more

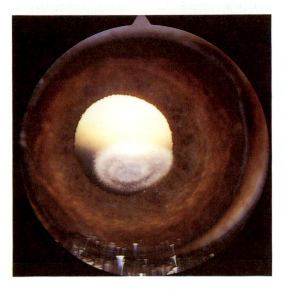

Figure 4.23 Crystalline stromal dystrophy in a 5 year old Shetland Sheepdog. Right eye.

severe manifestation of the condition with lipid deposition also occurring deeper in the cornea.

Corneal lipid deposition can occur secondarily to other primary coneoscleral diseases as a result of leakage of lipids from blood vessels. This is referred to as lipid keratopathy and may accompany conditions such as keratitis, episcleritis, or neoplasia, for example limbal melanoma, or occur as a sequence to cataract surgery. The appearance of the lipid deposit is variable; it may be a diffuse white color or appear as a granular deposit or as refractile 'flakes'. Lipid deposition as a circumferential ring in the paralimbal cornea is known as *arcus lipoides* and in such cases the possibility of predisposing systemic disease should be investigated. Deposited lipid crystals may occasionally erode through the corneal epithelium causing ulceration and pain. If the deposition is marked or progressive, the animal should be investigated for hyperlipoproteinemia and endocrinopathy.

Management of lipid keratopathy involves treatment for any underlying hyperlipoproteinemia and if the lesion is extensive, progressive or painful, a keratectomy may be required.

Calcareous degeneration is characterized by the presence of dense white often needle-shaped stromal deposits. These lesions frequently will ulcerate causing discomfort and may become vascularized. This condition affects older dogs and uremia may be a predisposing factor.

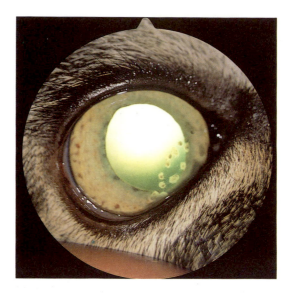

Figure 4.24   Keratic precipitates associated with toxoplasmosis in a 2 year old DSH cat. Right eye.

Keratectomy is indicated if the lesion causes discomfort or is extensive.

Corneal endothelial deposits

Inflammatory cells deposited as roundish, usually gray, foci on the corneal endothelial surface as a result of granulomatous anterior uveitis are known as keratic precipitates. They are more common in cats with anterior uveitis than in dogs and tend to be deposited inferiorly (Figure 4.24).

A slowly progressive thin pigment deposit involving the corneal endothelium and originating from the limbal region is sometimes observed and presumed to be due to migration or slow proliferation of limbal pigment.

Occasionally iris cysts (see below) rupture against the corneal endothelium leaving a donut-shaped deposit of pigment.

Alteration of corneal contour

A profound accumulation of fluid in the cornea may cause distortion of the corneal profile, an appearance which is referred to as keratoglobus. Other possible causes of misshapen corneal contour include corneal abscess and inclusion cyst, both of which are rare and necessitate keratectomy. Corneal abscesses consist of an accumulation of a pocket of grayish-white fluid within the cornea and are accompanied by conjunctival inflammation. Inclusion cysts are filled with a thick, white material and are associated with minimal inflammation although there are usually a few superficial blood vessels extending to them.

Deeper corneal ulcers will alter the corneal contour and when they extend down to Descemet's membrane may bulge forward as the result of the intraocular fluid pressure as a descemetocele (see p. 180–181). Healing of a corneal ulcer which has resulted in loss of corneal stroma may leave a corneal facet or an epithelialized indentation.

Corneal laceration, with or without iris prolapse, requires surgical repair of the wound, reformation of the anterior chamber and medical treatment to control possible infection and anterior uveitis.

The anterior chamber and anterior uvea

Congenital lesions of the iris include coloboma, persistent pupillary membranes, and iris cysts. Colobomas of the iris are rare, they may occur at the characteristic 6 o'clock position resulting in an irregular or false pupil. Persistent pupillary membranes are strands of iris tissue that can be single or multiple. They arise from the iris collarette and may be free floating or insert either onto the corneal endothelium, the iris, or the anterior lens capsule. Focal opacities of varying extent are associated with these insertions (see p. 97–98).

Anterior uveitis

Anterior uveitis is inflammation of the iris and ciliary body. Acute anterior uveitis is typically painful and is considered in Chapter 6. Animals with a low-grade chronic uveitis of insidious onset may be presented because the owner notices a change in the appearance of the eye rather than pain or discomfort. The potential etiologies of chronic uveitis are similar to those described for acute uveitis on p. 188–189 [14].

Clinical signs of chronic uveitis can include episcleral congestion, corneal changes (edema, vascularization, and deposition of keratic precipitates), deposition of inflammatory material in the anterior chamber, iris color changes, and lens changes. Typically the iris color changes consist of darkening with a loss of normal surface detail, although in some forms of uveitis such as the uveodermatological syndrome, there is iris depigmentation. A reddening of the iris (*rubeosis iridis*) may develop in animals with a light-colored iris, typically cats, and is due either to vascular engorgement or neovascularization. The inflammation may result in adhesions between the iris and the anterior capsule of the lens (posterior synechiae). These limit pupillary movement and often distort the pupil shape. Extensive posterior synechiae will block aqueous passage through the pupil forcing the iris to bulge anteriorly (iris bombé) and leading to a secondary glaucoma. The lens changes include pigment deposits on the anterior capsule due to transient adhesion of the iris to the lens capsule and cataract formation. Secondary lens luxation may occur, particularly in cats with feline immunodeficiency virus (FIV) induced uveitis. The uveo-dermatological syndrome (often erroneously referred to as the Vogt–Koyanagi–Harada syndrome or VKH) is a specific form of immune-mediated uveitis seen in dogs, most commonly the Arctic breeds. Anterior uveitis and a characteristic poliosis (whitening of the hair) and viteligo (depigmentation of the skin) around the eyes and muzzle are seen. Control of the uveitis is difficult and there is a serious risk of secondary glaucoma.

Blood-filled anterior chamber

Apart from inflammatory disease, hyphema may accompany systemic disease such as clotting disorders or hypertension, or may result from ocular disease such as chronic glaucoma, congenital lesions associated with persistence of embryonic blood vessels, neoplasia, retinal detachment, and trauma. There is a common association with preiridal fibrovascular membrane formation, or rubeosis irides; the new vessels on the iris surface are fragile and are frequently the source of spontaneous hyphema. Investigation of hyphema requires thorough

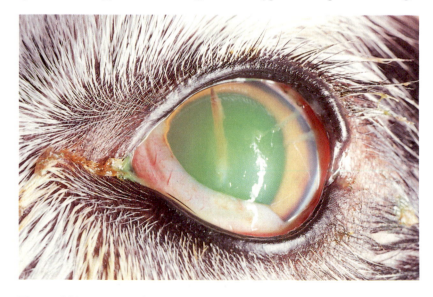

Figure 4.25   A linear foreign body (a thorn) and attendant anterior uveitis in a 4 year old crossbred dog. Left eye.

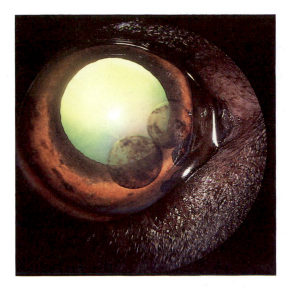

Figure 4.26   Multiple anterior uveal cysts demonstrating their appearance on transillumination in a 10 year old Doberman. Right eye.

ocular and systemic examination, ultrasonography (to investigate the possible presence of intraocular neoplasia), hematology, biochemistry, and blood pressure measurement. Non-specific treatment includes topical corticosteroids to control any concurrent uveitis.

Masses in the anterior chamber

Masses are readily visualized within the anterior chamber given adequate corneal transparency. Following uveitis, organized fibrin and other inflammatory product may be seen as strands or masses adherent to corneal endothelium, anterior lens capsule, or iris. Anterior chamber foreign bodies will be accompanied by corneal or scleral damage and a uveitic response (Figure 4.25). The iris cyst is typically a spherical, often free-floating structure of variable size in the anterior chamber (Figure 4.26), but on occasion its origin at the iridal pigment epithelium is indicated by a connecting strand. Usually such cysts are of no clinical significance although occasionally the size and number of them is such that vision may be obscured and removal by aspiration indicated. The presence of a luxated lens anterior to the iris (Figure 4.30) is usually heralded by a sudden onset glaucoma in the dog (see Chapter 6), but occasionally in this species and routinely in the cat the presence of the lens in the anterior chamber does not cause glaucoma.

Uveal tumors may be primary or secondary. The primary tumors include melanoma, adenoma, adenocarcinoma, and medulloepithe-

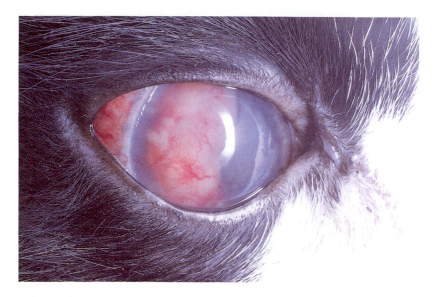

Figure 4.27   Ciliary adenocarcinoma involving the iris in an 8 year old DSH cat. Right eye.

lioma (Figure 4.27). The diagnosis of uveal neoplasia depends on the demonstration of a solid mass involving the iris or ciliary body, and histopathological confirmation is often not performed until the eye is enucleated. Most primary ocular tumors in the dog are benign but ultimately the eye will be destroyed by an accompanying uveitis or the resultant glaucoma. In an eye that is otherwise normal, owners may request local resection, although this is a skilled procedure and in many cases enucleation is eventually performed. Laser photocoagulation has been used to treat uveal tumors with some success and is likely to become more widely used in the future [15]. The commonest secondary uveal tumor is lymphoma, although any metastatic tumor embolus may locate in the eye. The ocular manifestations of lymphoma vary considerably and may not be specific for neoplasia; indeed anterior uveitis glaucoma, and/or intraocular hemorrhage may be the initial presenting feature [16]. For the treatment of secondary tumors, palliative enucleation, chemotherapy, or euthanasia of the terminal patient represent the treatment options.

Pupillary abnormalities

Ophthalmic patients may present with anisocoria, a difference in size between the two pupils. The clinician must determine which is the abnormal pupil, by comparing relative sizes in light and dark conditions, checking the direct and consensual light responses and performing visual tests. Possible causes of an abnormally dilated pupil include unilateral iris atrophy, glaucoma, oculomotor and parasympathetic nerve lesions, mydriatics, dysautonomia, severe unilateral retinal disease, optic neuropathy, and unilateral optic tract lesions. Causes of the unilaterally constricted pupil include anterior uveitis, synechiae, Horner's syndrome, miotics, and organophosphate poisoning. Cranial trauma may result in anisocoria and the prognosis is poor if this progresses to dilated non-responsive pupils. Where bilateral mydriasis or miosis is present the differential diagnosis should similarly consider all those causes listed for anisocoria.

The lens

Changes in the appearance of the lens most commonly result from a loss of transparency or because of its dislocation from its normal position. Gross opacification is readily discerned, but magnification and the use of slit-beam biomicroscopy are necessary to identify small lesions and to see which part of the lens is involved. Distant direct ophthalmoscopy makes it easy to differentiate between cataract and nuclear sclerosis. Cataract results in a black shadow against the reflection from the fundus whereas nuclear sclerosis presents no barrier to the fundus reflection. Nuclear sclerosis is a normal aging

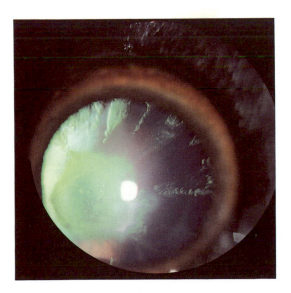

Figure 4.28 Posterior polar and equatorial cataract in a 7 year old Labrador Retriever. Left eye.

feature of the lens and is due to the compaction of the embryonic and fetal nuclear material. It has minimal effect on vision but the gray appearance of the lens often prompts a misdiagnosis of cataract. Lens opacity may be due to the attachment of posterior synechiae and any associated pigment migration, the presence of pupillary membranes, or the persistence of elements of the primary vitreous, but the commonest cause of opacity is cataract formation. Cataract is simply defined as an opacity of the lens and/or its capsule; there are a number of possible causes including genetic defects, congenital anomalies, diabetes mellitus, trauma, and as a result of other ocular conditions (e.g. uveitis, glaucoma, lens luxation, and retinal degeneration). With inherited cataract, the age of onset and the appearance of the opacity are often specific for the breed (Figures 4.28 and 4.29).

The reason for presentation of the cataract patient may be the abnormal appearance of the eye since the owner may be unaware of the degree of visual impairment. If the cataract is progressive or has a significant effect on vision then the patient should be assessed for suitability for surgery. This should involve complete systemic and ophthalmic examination together with electroretinography and ocular ultrasonography to determine if other ocular disease is present and to assess the integrity of the retina. There is no medical treatment for cataract but surgical extraction can successfully restore sight. Techniques currently employed include extracapsular lens extraction and phacoemulsification [17].

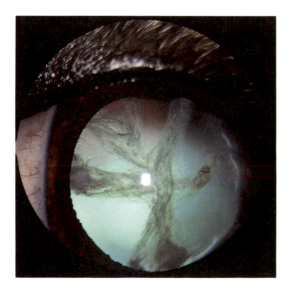

Figure 4.29 Cortical 'spoke wheel' cataract in a 9 year old Boston Terrier. Left eye.

Primary lens luxation most commonly occurs in the terrier breeds. The lens may move posteriorly into the vitreous cavity or, more commonly, anteriorly into or through the pupil (Figure 4.30). Its position within the pupil or the anterior chamber produces interference with the pupillary flow of aqueous and acute secondary glaucoma is the usual presenting feature (Chapter 6). Diagnosis is usually straightforward and the glaucoma should be relieved by osmotic diuretics followed by emergency lens extraction [18]. A posteriorly luxated lens does not necessarily require removal, although in some patients the lens repeatedly moves between the anterior chamber and the vitreous causing pain every time it is in the anterior chamber. Conservative long-term management is possible using long-acting miotics to maintain the lens within the vitreous cavity. Secondary lens luxation occurs in both cats and dogs as a result of conditions such as uveitis (particularly associated with FIV infection in cats), cataract formation, and glaucoma. Spontaneous lens luxation occurs infrequently in aged animals, but is rarely a cause of glaucoma. In most situations the extraction of the dislocated lens does not prove necessary.

The posterior segment

Leukocoria is defined as a white appearance to the pupil. The differential diagnoses include cataract, neoplasia, persistent hyper-

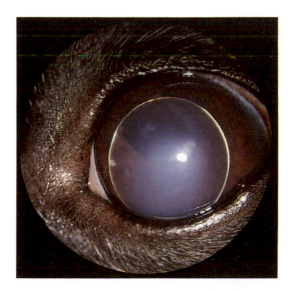

Figure 4.30 Primary anterior lens luxation in a 5 year old Jack Russell Terrier. Left eye.

plastic primary vitreous, vitreous abscess, posterior uveitis, and retinal detachment.

Persistent hyperplastic primary vitreous is a congenital cause of leukocoria in which posterior capsular and stromal fibrovascular plaques render the posterior lens opaque [19]. Cataract may also be present. The problem may be sporadic although it is inherited in some breeds notably the Doberman and Staffordshire Bull Terrier. The presence of retrolenticular vasculature is diagnostic although ocular ultrasonography may be needed to show the full extent of the involvement, particularly when cataract is present. Treatment is difficult because it involves the removal of the lens and the anterior vitreous.

Severe retinal dysplasia with retinal non-attachment or detachment may result in congenital leukocoria due to the presence of the retina against the posterior surface of the lens and often cataract formation. This condition is discussed further on p. 106–107.

Animals with bilateral retinal detachment will often present with blindness but, if the condition is unilateral and the retina is occupying the anterior vitreous or there is vitreal hemorrhage, the resulting abnormal appearance may be the reason for presentation [20]. Hypertensive retinopathy is now recognized commonly in older cats (Figure 4.31) and it may lead to retinal detachment and intraocular hemorrhage. Patients presenting with this problem should be investigated for cardiac, renal, and thyroid disease.

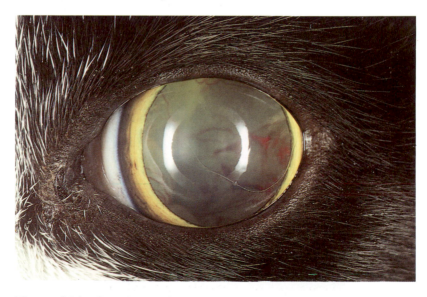

Figure 4.31 Complete retinal detachment resulting from hypertensive retinopathy associated with hyperthyroidism in a 13 year old DSH cat. Left eye.

Alterations in the quality of the tapetal reflex may be the reason for presentation. A 'glassy' appearance or 'glare' may be the layman's description of the pupil due to tapetal hyper-reflectivity following retinal degeneration or retinal detachment with disinsertion. The loss of the pupillary light response exacerbates the appearance. The funduscopic changes resulting from retinal degeneration are described on p. 110–112 and 146–153.

Generally the prognosis for vision in retinal detachment is poor due to late presentation of many of these cases. The treatment is discussed on p. 123.

REFERENCES

1. Dziezyc J, Hager DA and Millichamp NJ. Two-dimensional real-time ocular ultrasonography in the diagnosis of ocular lesions in dogs. *J. Am. Anim. Hosp. Ass.* 1987; **23**: 501–8.
2. Boydell P. Fine needle aspiration biopsy in the diagnosis of exophthalmos. *J. Small. Anim. Pract.* 1991; **32**: 542–6.
3. Gilger BC, Hamilton HL, Wilkie DA, Van der Woerdt A, McLaughlin SA and Whitley RD. Traumatic Proptosis in dogs and cats: 84 cases (1980–1993). *J. Am. Vet. Med. Ass.* 1995; **206**: 1186–90.
4. Bingaman DP, Lindley DM, Glickman NW Krohne SG and Bryan GM Intraocular gentamicin and glaucoma: a retrospective study in 60 dogs and cat eyes (1985–1993). *Vet. Comp. Ophthalmol* 1994; **4**: 113–9.
5. Kern TJ, Aromando MC and Erb HN. Horner's syndrome in dogs and cats: 100 cases (1975–1985). *J. Am. Vet. Med. Ass.* 1989; **195**: 369–73.
6. Gelatt KN and Gelatt JP. *Handbook of Small Animal Ophthalmic Surgery, Volume 1: Extraocular Procedures*, Oxford: Pergammon Press 1994: 98–104.
7. Johnson BW and Campbell KL. Dermatoses of the canine eyelid. *Compend. Contin. Educ. Pract. Vet.* 1989; **11**: 385–94.
8. Petersen-Jones SM. Repositioning prolapsed third eyelid glands while preserving secretory function. *In Pract.* 1991; **13**: 202–3.
9. Morgan RV, Duddy JM and McClurg K. Prolapse of the gland of the third eyelids in dogs: a retrospective study of 89 cases (1980 to 1990). *J. Am. Anim. Hosp. Ass.* 1993; **29**: 56–60.
10. Petersen-Jones SM. Differential diagnosis of the 'red eye' in small animals, *In Pract.* 1993; **15**: 55–64.
11. Startup FG. Corneal necrosis and sequestration in the cat: a review and record of 100 cases. *J. Small Anim. Pract.* 1988; **29**: 476–486.
12. Jackson PA, Kaswan RL, Merideth RE and Barrett PM Chronic superficial keratitis in dogs: a placebo-controlled trial of topical cyclosporine treatment. *Prog. Vet. Comp. Ophthalmol.* 1991; **1**: 269–75.
13. Crispin SM and Barnett KC. Dystrophy, degeneration and infiltration of the canine cornea. *J. Small Anim. Pract.* 1983; **24**: 63–83.
14. Crispin SM. Uveitis in the dog and cat. *J. Small Anim. Pract.* 1988; **29**: 429–47.

15. Nasisse MP, Davidson MG, Olivero DK, Brinkman M and Nelms S. Neodymium: YAG laser treatment of primary canine intraocular tumors. *Prog. Vet. Comp. Ophthalmol.* 1993; **3**: 152–7.
16. Krohne SG, Henderson NM, Richardson RC and Vestre WA. Prevalence of ocular involvement in dogs with multicentric lymphoma: prospective evaluation of 94 cases. *Vet. Comp. Ophthalmol.* 1994; **4**: 127–35.
17. Dziezyc J. Cataract surgery: current approaches. *Vet. Clin. North. Am. (Small Anim. Pract.)* 1990; **20**: 737–54.
18. Glover TL, Davidson MG, Nasisse MP and Olivero DK. The intracapsular extraction of displaced lenses in dogs: a retrospective study of 57 cases (1984–1990). *J. Am. Anim. Hosp. Ass.* 1995; **31**: 77–81.
19. Boevé MH, Stades FC, van der Linde-Sipman JS and Vrensen GFJM. Persistent hyperplastic tunica vasculosa lentis and primary vitreous (PHTVL/PHPV) in the dog: a comparative review. *Prog. Vet. Comp. Ophthalmol.* 1992; **2**: 163–72.
20. Hendrix DV, Nasisse MP, Cowen P and Davidson MG. Clinical signs, concurrent diseases and risk factors associated with retinal detachment in dogs. *Prog. Vet. Comp. Ophthalmol.* 1993; **3**: 87–91.

5
Visual Impairment

Kristina Narfström, Ellen Bjerkås and Björn Ekesten

EVALUATION OF VISUAL FUNCTION

This chapter deals with visual impairment and concerns diseases primarily related to the eyes, but also those occurring secondary to other systemic conditions. When an owner presents an animal with the complaint of visual impairment, careful questioning is of utmost importance and may often give an indication as to the nature of the disease. Essential questions are listed in Table 5.1.

Age

In a young animal, a congenital condition or malformation must be considered. Examples of infections in young animals are *ophthalmia neonatorum* in the dog and upper respiratory and ocular infection caused by feline herpesvirus-1 in the kitten. Degenerative diseases, like hereditary rod cone degeneration (generalized progressive retinal atrophy, PRA), and primary glaucomas most often develop in older animals.

Breed

A long list of diseases shows relation to breed, and knowledge of breed-specific diseases is of great importance. However, breed-related diseases show great variation in incidence in different parts of the world, which makes local knowledge essential. While, for example,

Table 5.1 Essential questions to ask

Age
Breed
General health
Other clinical signs
Onset (sudden or gradual)
Known etiology (i.e. injury, accident)
Initial clinical signs
Pain/no pain
Vision in daylight/poor light
Duration

primary glaucoma is a common disease in the American Cocker Spaniel in the USA, the condition is of less importance in this breed in northern Europe.

General health and other clinical signs

Visual impairment may occur as part of a systemic disease, and a general physical examination should always be performed. Examples of systemic diseases causing visual impairment are diabetes mellitus causing cataract, malignant lymphoma which may cause uveitis and retinal detachment, hypertension causing retinal hemorrhages and/or detachments and diseases affecting the central nervous system, impairing the condition or interpretation of the visual impulse.

Onset

The onset of impaired vision may be sudden, as in injuries, acute glaucoma, and certain inflammatory conditions, or occur gradually, as in chronic keratitis, most forms of cataracts and PRA. Injuries most often cause unilateral problems, while other conditions may be bilateral. In congenital conditions, the animal may have been born with reduced vision, or vision loss may occur secondarily. An example of the latter is retinal detachment or hemorrhage secondary to collie eye anomaly (CEA).

Known etiological factors

The owner is usually able to provide information when an eye has been injured. Useful information may also be vaccination status, as in corneal edema (blue eye) after vaccination with live modified hepatitus virus in dogs. A change in environment may impair an animal's immune balance. This is seen in cats with subclinical herpesvirus infection resulting in exacerbation of keratitis.

Initial clinical signs

Initial signs vary from some redness of the eye to acute vision loss. Early cases of keratoconjunctivitis sicca may show only moderate signs with conjunctivitis and mucoid discharge, while in chronic cases the corneas may suffer from infiltration of blood vessels and pigment deposits. In early stages of lens luxation, before the development of secondary intraocular diseases, clinical signs may be moderate with just some redness of the eye, while in acute uveitis the animal may show severe discomfort. One should remember that animals in their normal surroundings may apparently function more or less normally, even though visually impaired. Thus, the owner may not have noticed vision loss until the animal is introduced to an unfamiliar environment. A unilaterally blind animal often shows no noticeable evidence of blindness until the second eye becomes affected.

Pain

Assessment of pain may sometimes be difficult, as in certain cases of acute glaucoma. However, if a condition is painful, the animal will usually keep the eyelids closed and try to avoid examination. More subtle signs of pain or discomfort may be inappetence, lethargy, or otherwise altered behaviour. Most congenital conditions as well as retinal degenerations are not painful, while glaucoma, uveitis and perforating injuries may cause extreme pain. Cataracts are rarely painful, unless a lens-induced uveitis is present.

Vision in daylight and in dim light

This information is important when dealing with diseases of the retina. PRA, for example, causes initial night blindness, with a later reduction of day vision, while in sudden acquired retinal degeneration (SARD) both day and night vision are impaired simultaneously. Animals with cataracts in central parts of the lenses may show better vision in dim light than in broad daylight, due to pupil dilation.

Examination of the patient

General examination

This should be an assessment of the general condition including examination of circulation, respiration, mucous membranes, and peripheral lymph nodes. The owner should be questioned about appetite, thirst, and changes in the animal's behaviour. Information on the food should be obtained, as the animal's diet may have a bearing on its visual loss (cats fed dog food may develop a taurine-related retinopathy). Medication may influence the clinical signs; certain sulfonamides may be responsible for the development of keratoconjunctivitis sicca, and atropine drops impair pupillary light reflexes. In some cases laboratory workup is required.

Neurological examination

If a condition affecting the central nervous system is suspected, a full neurologic examination should be performed [1, 2]. Some causes of blindness of central nervous system (CNS) origin are given in Table 5.2. The general physical examination may already have revealed signs such as reduced vision, nystagmus, hearing loss, paresis of

Table 5.2   Some causes of blindness of CNS origin

Optic neuritis
Trauma to optic nerves
Hydrocephalus (juvenile or acute, decompensating)
Hepatic encephalopathy
Lysosomal storage diseases and other CNS degenerative diseases
Brain tumor (meningioma, lymphoma, pituitary, reticulosis)
Encephalitis (canine distemper, feline infectious peritonitis, toxoplasmosis)
Meningitis (bacterial, viral, fungal, or algal)
Cerebrosvascular accident (cats)
Brain trauma
Toxicity (lead, ivermectin, levamisole)
Parasites (migrating larvae)

face muscles, changes in behaviour or ataxia. A neurological examination should at least include testing of the cranial nerves, the
postural reactions, and the spinal reflexes. Cranial nerves II (optic)
and III (oculomotor) affect the pupillary light reflexes, and III, IV
(trochlear), and VI (abducent) determine ocular movements. The
trigeminal nerve (V) contains sensory fibers from the cornea and the
skin of the face, while the facial nerve (VII) is responsible for the
motor function of the facial muscles including the eyelids. The
trigeminal and facial nerves are tested together by tapping or pricking
each side of the face. A sympathetic nerve which leaves the spinal
cord in the cervicothoracic region is responsible for pupil dilatation
and for the tone of the smooth muscles in the periorbital fascia and
eyelids (Müller muscles).

Testing vision

Obstacle course

The easiest way of testing an animal's vision is to set up an obstacle
course in unfamiliar surroundings and carefully observe the animal's
movements through the area. The test should be performed both in
normal and in dim light to assess day (photopic) and night (scotopic)
vision. An obstacle course can be set up with almost anything. A set
of small buckets put upside down can be moved around to create new
paths. A normal animal learns the path after one or two attempts,
which may lead the examiner to draw the wrong conclusions. It may
be noted that dogs with reduced vision tend to use their nose more
eagerly, whereas cats tend to feel with their paws.

Cotton ball

An additional way of vision testing is to hold up a cotton ball, attract the animal's attention to it, and then drop the ball. The ball may be dropped both in front of the animal and to its sides to assess central and peripheral vision. Most animals will follow the movement of the cotton ball. However, puppies, lethargic animals, and some cats may show little interest in the procedure. These animals may be tested by dragging a noiseless object, like a cotton ball tied to a thread, along the floor. If not too lethargic, the animal will want to have a closer look at the object.

Swinging light

In a darkened room the examiner watches for corresponding head or eye movements while the light beam from a penlight is swept across the visual axis in various planes. Visual field defects are difficult to assess in animals, but an attempt can be made by repeating the procedures with one eye blindfolded.

The optic nerve

The optic nerve is the afferent path both for vision and pupillary light reflexes. In the cat and dog, about two-thirds of the optic nerve fibers cross in the optic chiasm to the opposite side of the brain. In the optic tract, 80% of the nerve fibers project via the lateral geniculate nucleus to the visual cortex of the cerebrum, whereas 20% go to the midbrain. The midbrain structures handle reflex vision, like dazzle reflex and pupillary light reflexes, and also visual input for balance and gaze fixation.

Normal function of the optic nerve can be tested in many ways. Practical testing includes:

- The menace reaction
- The visual placing reaction
- The pupillary light reflexes
- The dazzle reflex

Note the difference between reactions and reflexes: a reaction involves higher (cortical) function, whereas reflexes are not dependent upon cortical function and may be normal in an animal with abnormal vision perception associated with higher lesions.

The menace reaction

A normal menace reaction requires a normal visual pathway (the sensory pathway), as well as a normal facial nerve, the motor pathway (Figure 5.1).

The visual pathway consists of the retina, the optic nerve, the optic chiasm, the optic tract, the lateral geniculate nucleus in the thalamus,

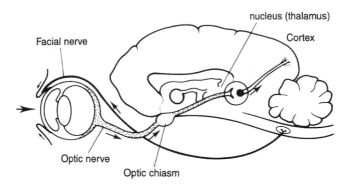

Figure 5.1   The menace reaction. A sudden movement in front of the eye produces a rapid blink. The menace reaction requires normal visual pathways to the visual cortex as well as normal motor pathways to the eyelids.

the optic radiation, and the visual cortex. The motor pathway involves the connection from the visual cortex to the facial nucleus and the facial nerve (VII).

The menace reaction is a way of testing if the animal is visual, as a positive response (inherited by a blink) tells that an image has been formed in the visual cortex. The animal is threatened by bringing a hand over the eye from out of the visual field or to open a clenched fist in front of the eye without causing air currents to stimulate hairs or cornea. It is, however, important to note that the menace reaction can be absent in animals with cerebellar or facial nerve lesions, without the animal being blind, and that seriously ill animals may react poorly to the stimulus.

The visual placing reactions

Normal visual placing reactions require normal visual pathways to the cerebral cortex, communication from the visual cortex to the motor cortex, and motor pathways to the lower motor neurones (final common pathway) of the forelimbs.

Testing in small dogs and cats can be performed by holding the animal in front of a table. The animal is allowed to see the table surface when moved towards the edge of the table. Normal animals reach for the surface before the carpus touches the table. Some cats and dogs that are accustomed to being held may ignore the table and animals with neurologic deficits may perform the test poorly. Peripheral visual fields can be tested by making a lateral approach to the table. Larger dogs can be led over a curb or a step.

The dazzle reflex

This is a stimulation of the optic nerve by suddenly shining a bright light into the eye. Normally, this will make the animal blink. The dazzle reflex (or the retinal light reflex) is not a reaction, that is, it is subcortical, mediated by reflex centers in the midbrain with fibers to the facial nucleus.

The pupillary light reflexes

Most important in the evaluation of visual function is the assessment of the pupillary light reflexes (PLR) (Figure 5.2). The afferent, or sensory pathway, involves the retina, the optic nerve (II) and the optic chiasm to the optic tract, where the majority of the fibers continue the

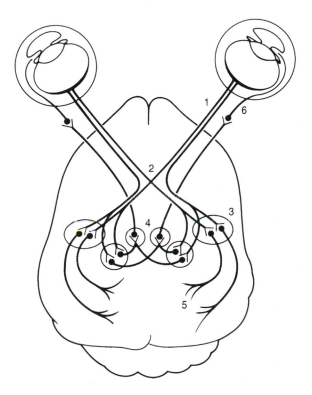

Figure 5.2 The pupillary light reflex arc. Shining light into one eye produces constriction of the pupil in the stimulated eye (direct pupillary light reflex) as well as in the contralateral eye (indirect pupillary light reflex). 1, optic nerve (II); 2, optic chiasm; 3, lateral geniculate nucleus; 4, parasympathetic nucleus of CN III (Edinger–Westphal) nucleus; 5, visual cortex; 6, oculomotor nerve (III).

visual pathway to the lateral geniculate nucleus. However, about 20% leave the optic tract before the lateral geniculate body and course towards the midbrain, where they synapse in the pretectal nuclei. From the pretectal nuclei, fibers are distributed to the parasympathetic nuclei of the oculomotor (III) nerve (the Edinger–Westphal nuclei). The efferent or motor pathway extends via the parasympathetic fibers of the cranial nerve III through the ciliary ganglion to the ciliary body and iris sphincter muscle.

At the optic chiasm, optic nerve fibers decussate to different degrees amongst species. As a rule, the more lateral the eyes are placed in the skull, the greater the degree of decussation. In the dog and cat, about two-thirds of the optic nerve fibers cross in the optic chiasm to the opposite side of the brain. Temporal nerve fibers from the nasal visual field remain uncrossed in the optic tract on the same side, while nasal fibers from the temporal visual field cross to the opposite optic tract. This knowledge is important when assessing visual field defects in humans, but of less importance in animals, where visual field defects are difficult to evaluate.

Pupillary constriction and dilation is essentially a balance between parasympathetic and sympathetic control. The constrictor muscle of the iris, innervated by the parasympathetic fibers of the oculomotor nerve (III), is a sphincter muscle located at the pupillary border and is more powerful than the dilator muscle, which runs along the iris in a radial fashion. The dilator muscle is innervated by sympathetic nerves. These nerves leave the spinal cord in the cervicothoracic region and run along the neck in the vagosympathetic trunk, through the middle ear cavity and through the superior orbital fissure before entering the eye. When evaluating anisocoria, it must be remembered that since sympathetics dilate the pupils, a sympathetic lesion will be most noticeable in the dark, as a small pupil stays small. Conversely, the parasympathetics constrict the pupils. Therefore, in parasympathetic lesions, as the pupil stays dilated, the difference in pupillary size will be greater in the light.

Before testing the pupillary light reflexes, it is important to evaluate the size of both pupils, and to note any difference in pupil size – anisocoria. A dim light is directed from below and any changes in pupil size noted. Remember that an anxious or excited animal may have widely dilated pupils due to sympathetic stimulation, and that re-evaluation of pupil size after the animal has relaxed may be necessary. Reflexes in young animals may be sluggish and incomplete, probably related to maturational myelination of the optic nerve.

Testing of direct and consensual pupillary light reflexes

In a darkened room, a bright light is shone into one eye. Normally this causes a rapid and complete pupillary constriction in the stimulated eye, the *direct* PLR. The constriction in the other eye, the consensual (or *indirect*) PLR, is slightly slower. The indirect PLR is produced because of decussation of nerve fibers in the optic chiasm as well as the synapsing of fibers from both sides in the nuclei of the midbrain. By evaluating the direct and consensual PLRs it is possible to localize defects along the reflex arcs, as well as evaluating the function of the retina and optic nerve in an eye with large lesions in the anterior structures.

The PLRs are independent of cortical vision but still provide useful information on the integrity of the components of the afferent and efferent pathways. As the pupillary light reflexes do not involve higher (cortical) structures, a positive reflex does not necessarily mean that the animal has normal vision.

It may be noted that blindness with an abnormal PLR localizes the lesion rostral to the lateral geniculate body, while blindness with a normal PLR reveals the lesion to involve the lateral geniculate body, optic radiation, or visual cortex.

Reflex vision

Reflex vision is mediated in the midbrain and may be tested by

- The vestibulo–ocular reflex (Doll's eye reflex)
- The tonic neck and eye reflexes

The Doll's eye reflex is tested by moving the animal's head from side to side while observing the eye movements. Normally, the animal will produce rapid eye movements as compensation for the head movements to maintain clear vision. This reflex involves both the visual and vestibular pathways, but vestibular pathways predominate and will produce these movements even in the absence of vision.

The tonic neck and eye reflexes serve to maintain the original direction of vision and head position. The reflex is tested by standing the animal on all four legs and flexing and extending the neck to extremes. As the neck is extended, the eyes maintain their forward gaze, but the forelegs extend and the hindlegs flex. The reverse happens when the neck is flexed.

Refraction

The optical properties of the eye probably play an important role in visual discrimination in small animals, as well as in people. Refractive errors, e.g. myopia and hyperopia, are known to exist in dogs [3]. Although refractive errors sometimes may be suspected from the behaviour of the patient, the refractive state of the eye can be objectively determined using a retinoscope and a lens bar in animals. The technique is called retinoscopy or skiascopy. Retinoscopy is easily performed in most dogs and cats after instillation of a topical cyclo-plegic. Contact lenses, which correct for the refractive error and therefore increase the performance of the patient, can be used to verify the diagnosis. Long-term use of contact lenses to correct refractive errors is usually expensive in small animals, as retention is somewhat problematic.

Electrophysiology

Electrophysiological testing becomes invaluable in animals with visual dysfunction [4, 5]. Different procedures can be performed depending on the site of a suspected lesion, such as the retina, optic nerve, or the visual cortex. To examine visual function clinically, the recording of two types of response is recommended. One reflects the retina, the electroretinogram (ERG), the other reflects the brain, the visual evoked potential (VEP). The ERG allows a rapid and objective examination of the outer and inner retina while the VEP depends on normal optic nerve function and therefore reflects the conduction of the retinal signal to the brain. Because the area centralis region is magnified in the optic nerve and brain response, the VEP also provides some insight into potential visual acuity.

ERG

The ERG is a technique for observing the changes of electrical potential that occur when the eye is stimulated by light. These voltage changes, generated in the retina, reflect the responses of several classes of cell summed across the retina. They are critically dependent on the function of the retinal photoreceptors, i.e. the rods and cones. The ERG is usually recorded by means of a corneal contact lens electrode in response to a defined flash of light or repeated flashes (flicker) and displayed on an oscilloscope or on a computer screen. General anesthesia, intubation, and continuous monitoring of the patient is recommended during the procedure.

In veterinary ophthalmology ERG has mainly two broad applica-tions: the easiest and most straightforward simply tests whether or not a standard stimulus elicits an ERG response under a specific lighting condition. An example of this application is in an animal with complete cataracts. An ERG is indicated before proceeding to catar-act surgery in order to ascertain that the retina is functional and not affected by PRA. The second and more sophisticated application is the study of rod and cone function as part of research projects or in the early diagnosis of hereditary retinal dystrophies.

A complex set of processes, PI, PII, and PIII, first described by Granit in 1933 [6], collectively comprise the ERG response, with its a-, b- and in some types of recordings, c-waves. Grossly, the a-wave reflects the membrane current of photoreceptors and thus reflects their activity directly. The b-wave is generated as a complicated interaction, involving potassium movement between the bipolar and Müller cells, in response to input from the photoreceptors. The c-wave, is generated mainly through hyperpolarization of the apical membrane of the pigment epithelium and thus reflects retinal pigment epithelial cell function.

The rod photoreceptors mainly function under scotopic conditions, and the cones mainly under photopic conditions. ERG recordings thus represent various combinations of rod and cone responses depending on the specific lighting used as background and/or stimulus. Therefore, it is of utmost importance that a fixed protocol is used to obtain meaningful ERGs. In order to interpret the ERG responses successfully it is, moreover, recommended that a technique be used that allows for the direct separation of rod and cone contributions to the ERG [7, 8].

The waveform of the ERG together with the amplitude and implicit times of the a- and b-waves are most often used when evaluating ERGs in a clinical situation. Comparisons are made of the observed responses to those of normals or controls. It should be noted that there are species, breed, and age-related variations in ERG parameters so comparisons have always to be made with breed and age-matched animals.

VEP

Using active scalp electrodes VEPs can be recorded in anesthetized animals using stroboscopic flashes of light and averaging techniques [9]. VEPS are cone dominated and reflect activity in a small part of the central area of the retina. Fibers from the central area of the retina are projected onto the surface of the occipital cortex, whereas fibers from the peripheral areas are projected to deeper parts of the cortex and are not readily recorded. Apart from the central area of the retina, VEP mainly tests function of the postretinal structures such as the optic nerve and the visual cortex.

The waveform of the VEP consists of three major positive waves, the P1, P2, and P3. The characteristics of the VEP recording depend on a complex array of spatial and temporal conditions of light stimulation including luminance, contrast, and rate of stimulation. Depth of consciousness, age, visual acuity, and degree of light adaptation also influence the VEP.

The VEP is currently used mainly for research purposes, but the technique certainly has evolving clinical applications in the assessment of disease affecting the optic nerve and central visual systems. VEPs and ERGs can, moreover, be recorded simultaneously in the anesthetized animal, which makes it possible to evaluate visual function electrophysiologically in a more complete fashion.

CONGENITAL DISEASE AND MALFORMATIONS

Anophthalmia, nanophthalmia, and microphthalmia

In anophthalmia, the globe is more or less absent. This is a rare condition caused by a defect in the formation of the optic vesicle from the neuro ectoderm. Histologic examination of orbital tissue may reveal traces of rudimentary optic structures.

Microphthalmia is relatively common in the dog, and may present as a small but otherwise normal globe. This form of microphthalmia is termed nanophthalmia. The term microphthalmia, however, is usually used to describe a small and abnormal globe, the result of retarded or aberrrant development of the optic vesicle. The associated ocular anomalies, include retinal dysplasia, malformations of the lens, and developmental tissue defects (colobomas).

Microphthalmia is seen more frequently in certain breeds, including the Collie breeds, English Cocker Spaniel, and Dobermann Pinscher, but may occur spontaneously in dogs of any breed. Teratogenic agents as well as hereditary factors may cause malformations of the eyes. Microphthalmia may occur uni- or bilaterally, and one or more littermates may be affected.

Clinical findings

Anophthalmic or grossly microphthalmic eyes should not be difficult to recognize. Mild cases of microphthalmia or nanophthalmia may cause diagnostic problems, especially if the condition occurs bilaterally. In certain breeds, like the Collie and the Shetland Sheepdog, the breed standard demands small eyes, making differentiation between normal and microphthalmic eyes difficult. The following features may be of help when comparing a unilaterally microphthalmic eye to its fellow normal eye. Compare both eyes by inspection from above and in front of the animal and observe differences in the palpebral fissure, the eye being recessed into the orbit (enophthalmia) and/or protrusion of the third eyelid. Note the exposure of the sclera and the diameter of the cornea, as the majority of microphthalmic eyes present with a smaller than normal cornea (microcornea). Closer examination may reveal abnormalities including persistent pupillary membranes, abnormal pupillary (dyscoria), cataracts and multifocal retinal dysplasia or retinal detachment. Colobomas may be present, but are more rarely diagnosed. There are often abnormal eye movements such as a 'searching' nystagmus or a fine oscillatory nystagmus.

Differential diagnosis

Difference in pigmentation between two otherwise normal eyes is not uncommon and should not be confused with abnormalities of the eyes. Phthisis bulbus (shrinkage of the eye) occurs as a result of severe trauma or as an end-stage of intraocular inflammation. This condition is commonly preceded by a history of red eye and ocular pain, whereas microphthalmia is painless. Microphthalmia as a congenital condition is usually detected in the young animal, while phthisis bulbus may occur in animals of any age.

Prognosis and treatment

Abnormal development of the eye cannot be treated and the prognosis depends on the degree of visual impairment and whether the condition is uni- or bilateral. Secondary cataracts may develop and chronic conjunctivitis due to poor configuration of eyelids and globe may need daily irrigation. Cataract surgery in these eyes is unlikely to be rewarding. Enucleation may be recommended if the microphthalmic eye is blind and causes discomfort to the animal. The use of the animal for future breeding is not advised, particularly in the breeds where the condition is suspected to be inherited.

Persistent pupillary membranes (PPM)

During the embryonal phase the future pupil is covered by a vascular membrane, the pupillary membrane. This membrane is formed during development of the eye by anastomoses between the *tunica vasculosa lentis*, which branches from the hyaloid artery and forms a meshwork around the lens, and vascular loops from the annular vessel in front of the lens. Normally, the pupillary membrane begins to regress about 2 weeks before birth and has completely disappeared by 2 to 4 weeks after birth. Small remnants of the membrane are frequent in animals and of no significance. These may be seen as strands on the iris or as thin threads hanging from the surface of the iris. Larger persisting parts of the membrane may cause visual impairment. The remnants may extend across the pupil, to the lens or to the cornea, or both. Where attached to the lens, there may be cataract formation, and attachment to the corneal endothelium may cause focal corneal scarring or edema. Very small remnants may also be seen as pigmented flecks on the anterior lens capsule.

Clinical findings

PPM is congenital and may therefore be diagnosed in the young animal. The condition is not painful and there is no history of previous injury to the eye. With corneal involvement, the opacity does not stain with fluorescein. A genetic disposition has been described in the Basenji and has been suggested in the English Cocker Spaniel and the Collie [10, 11]. More than one puppy in a litter may be affected.

Treatment and prognosis

There is no effective treatment for this congenital condition, but unless the changes are extensive, vision is not affected. Affected dogs from breeds where a hereditary disposition is suspected should not be used for breeding.

Congenital lens disorders

These disorders are usually part of other developmental abnormalities of the eye and may be due to a chance error in embryogenesis. In some cases, however, the abnormalities have a hereditary background.

Congenital developmental abnormalities of the lens, which often occur in combination with other malformations of the eye, such as persistence of the hyaloid system or microphthalmia, include:

- Aphakia – the total absence of the lens or the presence of rudimentary parts of the lens. This is a rare condition.
- Microphakia – inadequate size of the lens. Elongated ciliary processes will be seen surrounding the lens, and the lens borders are clearly visible when the pupil is dilated. The condition may be breed related, as in the Miniature Schnauzer, where it is associated with congenital cataract.
- Spherophakia – an abnormal spherical shape to the lens which is usually microphakic as well.
- Coloboma – where the lens has an equatorial notching (Figure 5.3). The zonular fibers are either deficient or absent in this area. This condition is usually associated with congenital cataract and colobomas of the iris and ciliary body.
- Lenticonus/lentiglobus – a thinning of the lens capsule permitting the cortex to bulge, causing a conical malformation at the anterior or, most commonly, the posterior pole. Lentiglobus is more severe than lenticonus. The capsule in the affected area may show dysplastic or degenerative changes which will influence lens metabolism and result in a cataract. The abnormality is most often diagnosed in connection with abnormalities of the posterior hyaloid system, as described in persistent hyperplastic tunica vasculosa lentis/persistent hyperplastic primary vitreous (PHTVL/PHPV) in the Dobermann Pinscher [12], or in connection with microphthalmia and secondary cataract. A congenital defect of the lens including cataract, posterior lenticonus, and sometimes also

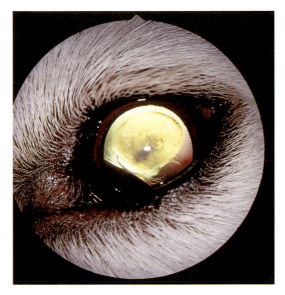

Figure 5.3 Congenital malformations of the lens in a 1 year old Samoyed dog: unilateral lens coloboma and cataract.

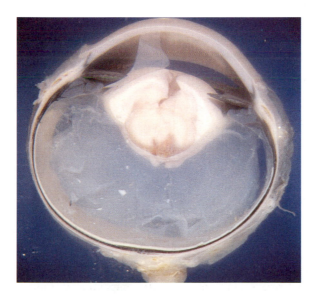

Figure 5.4 Posterior lenticonus, with rupture of the posterior lens capsule, in the eye illustrated, and bilateral congenital cataract in a 12 week old Cavalier King Charles Spaniel dog.

microphthalmia has been described in the Cavalier King Charles Spaniel (Figure 5.4) [13].

- Cataracts–nuclear and sometimes posterior and/or anterior cortical opacification with or without capsular involvement is sporadically observed in litters of several breeds. This type of congenital cataract has been described specifically in the English Cocker Spaniel [11]. In the West Highland White Terrier a specific type of posterior suture line cataract has been described as well as congenital complete cataracts [14].

Persistent hyaloid artery (PHA)

The hyaloid artery is present in fetal life, but will normally undergo regression during the first postnatal weeks. Remnants of the obliterated hyaloid artery which persist without any other abnormalities are referred to as PHA [15]. The artery can remain as a cord, still containing blood, between the optic disc and the lens. Usually, however, only a small connective tissue strand remains.

Clinical findings

The persistent hyaloid artery can be seen as a white strand adherent to the posterior lens capsule, below the posterior pole, stretching back into the vitreous body and moving with the eye movements. Occasionally, the hyaloid vessel arises from an anomalous superficial retinal vessel. Small vessel remnants do not affect vision, but at the site of adherence to the lens there may be a focal opacity (Mittendorf's dot). Secondary cataracts may develop in this area. The condition may occur uni- or bilaterally and is occasionally seen in the dog. A familial disposition has been suspected in the Sussex Spaniel.

Persistent hyperplastic tunica vasculosa lentis/persistent hyperplastic primary vitreous (PHTVL/PHPV)

In this disorder, parts of the hyaloid system and primitive vitreous become hyperplastic and remain postnatally instead of undergoing normal regression [12, 16]. Embryologic alterations occur in the eye cup, the primary vitreous, the hyaloid artery, and the *tunica vasculosa lentis*. The hyperplasia and lack of normal regression are considered to be caused by a disharmony between growth factors and inhibitors within the eye. In severe cases, secondary cataracts develop. The condition may be uni- or bilateral and may occur sporadically in any animal. In the Dobermann Pinscher primarily, but also in other breeds such as the Staffordshire Bull Terrier [17], the disorder occurs bilaterally and appears to be inherited by an incomplete dominant mode of inheritance.

Clinical findings

In the mildest form of PHTVL/PHPV, very small dots of residual tissue from the vascular network are found retrolental on the posterior lens capsule. These dots do not change further and do not influence vision. They are only seen by use of a slit-lamp biomicroscope, and may be difficult to diagnose in puppies because of small eye size. PHTVL may also be seen as vascular loops anterior to the lens. The severe forms occur bilaterally and often leads to visual impairment. A plaque of white fibrovascular tissue can remain on the posterior capsule, accompanied by retrolental dots. In addition, larger parts of the hyaloid system can persist and may be accompanied by pigment or blood in the lens, lenticonus, or other lens malformations (Figures 5.5 and 5.6). Secondary cataracts develop in the most severe forms, either present at birth or occurring in juvenile life.

Diagnosis and differential diagnosis

The condition is congenital and can be diagnosed in the puppy. A division into degrees, depending on the severity of the disorder, has been suggested. The disease does not include persistent pupillary membranes as described earlier, but small loops of the *tunica vasculosa lentis* system may be seen adjacent to the anterior capsule of the

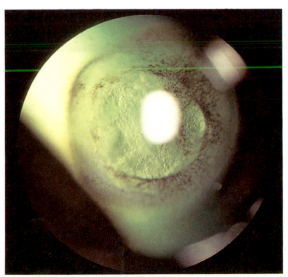

Figure 5.5 PHTVL/PHPV in a 9 month old Dobermann Pinscher. Fibrovascular tissue and pigmentation are seen on the posterior lens capsule as well as posterior lenticonus.

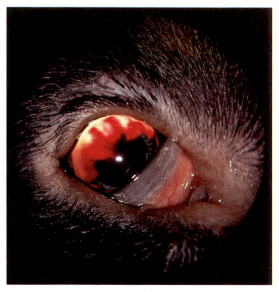

Figure 5.6   Intralenticular bleeding and low-grade uveitis is seen in conjunction with PHTVL/PHPV in this 1 year old Dobermann Pinscher.

lens. Differential diagnosis includes primary cataract or retinal detachment.

Therapy and prognosis

In severely abnormal eyes, lens extraction (see cataract therapy) can be performed together with vitrectomy. The prognosis for the operation is less favorable than in uncomplicated extracapsular lens extraction, because of the increased incidence of intra- and postoperative complications. Examination of Dobermann Pinscher puppies at about 7 weeks of age is recommended. Affected animals should not be used for breeding.

Congenital vitreous opacification

Vitreous opacification is uncommon and is usually due to hemorrhage associated with congenital retinal abnormalities. These may result from tearing of blood vessels in a detached retina or from retinal neovascularization.

The congenital diseases most commonly connected with blood in the vitreous are:

- Collie Eye Anomaly (CEA) in the Collie breeds. The hemorrhage usually occurs sporadically in the young dog, most often before two years of age.

- Total retinal dysplasia or non-attachment as seen sporadically in many breeds, and as an inherited condition in the Labrador Retriever, Sealyham Terrier, Bedlington Terrier, and occasionally the English Springer Spaniel.
- Multiple congenital ocular anomalies, as may be seen after mating of two merle-colored dogs and in the Australian Shepherd dog.
- Other conditions including preretinal arteriolar loops and vascular malformations.

Clinical findings

Hemorrhage in the vitreous is diagnosed uni- or bilaterally as blood seen behind the lens. The blood may also pass forward into the anterior segment of the eye. The condition is not usually painful.

Diagnosis

Examination of the fellow eye, if unaffected, may reveal congenital anomalies of types that may cause vitreous hemorrhage. The breed incidence is also important to consider.

Differential diagnosis

Intralenticular hemorrhage may be seen in connection with PHTVL/PHPV. The hemorrhage in this disorder, however, is within the retrolental plaque of tissue and sometimes also within the lens (Figure 5.6). Breed incidence must be considered.

Hyphema (blood in the anterior chamber) may resemble vitreous hemorrhage, and may occur from the same disorder (CEA), but will most often represent a different condition, like trauma, uveitis, or neoplasia.

Hyperviscosity is usually associated with monoclonal gammopathies. A thorough clinical examination should be performed. This disease, however, is usually diagnosed in older animals.

Treatment and prognosis

Surgical removal (vitrectomy) of congenital intravitreal hemorrhage is not recommended. The condition is serious because it usually indicates a severe disorder of the posterior segment. This is especially true if the blood remains unclotted, as this indicates continuing bleeding. The hemorrhage may seemingly clear if the dog is inactive for a period, but will return as soon as the dog is exercised. If, however, the hemorrhage should clear permanently, the vitreous may undergo degenerative changes which may lead to traction of the retina with subsequent detachment. More uncommonly, secondary glaucoma or uveitis may develop.

Congenital malformations of the retina and the optic nerve

The retina can be congenitally malformed in several ways including involvement of all layers of the neuroretina, such as in retinal dysplasia, or affecting specific cells in the retina, such as rod–cone dysplasia or retinal pigment epithelial cell dystrophy. In certain defects structures posterior to the retina are malformed as well as retinal structures, in posterior segment colobomata. Congenital malformations are often caused by hereditary factors but some are also induced by infection or x-irradiation, such as retinal dysplasia (see below), or may occur as a spontaneous malformation. See Table 5.3 for a summary of hereditary retinal disease affecting specific cells of the neurosensory retina in the dog and cat.

General treatment

There is usually no effective treatment for congenital malformations of the posterior segment of the eye. If the defect is known to be hereditary, preventive measures need to be taken in the breeding program. The rule of thumb is not to use affected individuals for breeding. Breeders are also recommended not to use known carriers of the defect in their breeding, as for example the parents of an affected animal and the affected animal's off-spring in an autosomal recessive disorder.

Retinal dysplasia (RD)

RD and multifocal RD (retinal folds) are ocular anomalies caused by an intrinsic abnormality of neural retinal differentiation [18]. Morphology shows a detached (or non-attached) retina, or folding and rosette formation of the neuronal retinal cells, respectively. The disease is believed to be inherited as an autosomal recessive trait in the breeds of dog that have been described genetically so far. Retinal dysplasia (complete type) has been described in e.g. the Sealyham and Bedlington Terrier breeds, the Labrador Retreiver, the Australian Shepherd dog and the English Springer Spaniel. Dogs affected with multifocal RD include the Labrador Retriever, American Cocker Spaniel, English Springer Spaniel, Beagle, Cavalier King Charles Spaniel, Rottweiler, and the Golden Retriever. Multifocal RD has also been observed in the cat.

Clinical findings

The ophthalmoscopic appearance is typical. In complete RD most or all of the neuroretina is detached (or non-attached). In multifocal RD, vermiform streaks or spots are seen typically around the retinal blood vessels dorsal to the optic disc. The lesions are most often bilateral

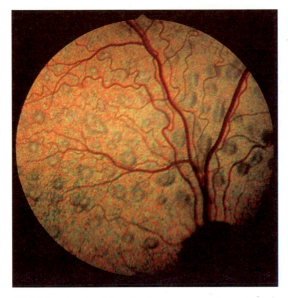

Figure 5.7 Multifocal retinal dysplasia may sometimes be severe and cause reduction in visual capacity as seen in this 4 year old English Springer Spaniel.

but the extent of the retinal changes may vary between the eyes. In complete RD the animal is most often blind while in multifocal RD vision is usually unaffected. Nystagmus may be present in blind puppies. Cataracts and skeletal abnormalities in conjunction with RD have been described in the homozygously affected Labrador retriever.

Specific treatment and prognosis

Therapy is not effective. Blindness is permanent in eyes with detached neural retinas and affected eyes may develop neovascular glaucoma and intraocular hemorrhage. Euthanasia is recommended in bilaterally affected puppies. In multifocal RD vision is often unaffected and will most often stay so throughout life. An exception is multifocal RD in the Springer Spaniel in which slowly progressive multifocal atrophic areas of the retina can result in severe visual impairment (Figure 5.7).

Secondary RD

Abnormal retinal differentiation with formation of retinal folds and rosettes occurs spontaneously in dogs and cats. Causes may be maternal infections, intrauterine trauma, vitamin A deficiency during pregnancy, irradiation, and idiopathic. Clinical signs are similar to those above. Other ocular signs often accompany the secondary type of retinal dysplasia such as cataracts, uveitis, and synechia formation.

Optic nerve hypoplasia and aplasia

This refers to an abnormal differentiation of the ganglion cell and nerve fiber layers of the retina resulting in a paucity of axons in the optic nerve and optic chiasm. This uncommon condition is either uni- or bilateral. Histologically it is seen as a reduction in the number of ganglion cells and thinning of the nerve fiber layer in the retina. The defect has been reported in several breeds and believed to be hereditary in some [19, 20].

Clinical findings

The clinical findings depend on the severity of the defect. If bilateral, the animal is usually blind but if unilateral the problem is often not noticed by the owner. The pupils are typically dilated and the pupillary light reflexes are non-functional. In cases of unilateral hypoplasia the affected eye may still show an indirect (or consensual) response. Ophthalmoscopically the disc is abnormally small and dark, often gray in appearance.

Treatment

There is no treatment except preventive measures in breeding in cases of a suspected hereditary background. Affected individuals should therefore not be used for breeding.

Posterior segment colobomas

A coloboma is a congenital tissue defect manifested by a pit, hole, fissure, or notch. A posterior segment coloboma may affect the overlying tissue such as neural retina, choroid, and sclera and often affects the optic disc. Colobomas in the Collie breeds are part of the Collie eye anomaly complex and hereditary optic disc colobomas have been reported in the Basenji dog. In cats colobomas of the choroid have been described with a hereditary background and may be seen associated with eyelid agenesis. Very extensive colobomas may cause blindness, while small ones cause no obvious visual problems.

Collie eye anomaly (CEA)

CEA is a common defect with a frequency over 90% in the Rough Collie in the USA 25–30 years ago. The prevalence in Scandinavia

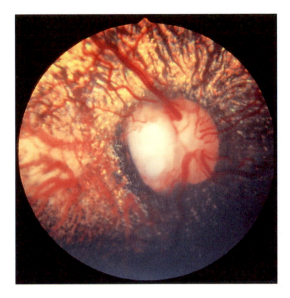

Figure 5.8   Choroidal hypoplasia and coloboma of the optic nerve head, as seen in this young Collie, are signs of Collie Eye Anomaly (CEA).

today is much lower, at about 40%. The disease is a congenital inherited ocular anomaly of the dog, which is suggested to be inherited as a simple autosomal recessive trait [21]. Etiologic factors include the failure of normal closing of the fetal fissure during development of the eye. The defect results in bilateral changes of variable severity that may affect the retina, choroid, sclera and/or the optic disc [22]. The essential lesion is choroidal hypoplasia which may or may not be accompanied by other defects (Figure 5.8). Affected breeds are the Rough and Smooth Collie, Shetland Sheepdog, Australian Shepherd, and the Border Collie.

Clinical findings and significance

Funduscopic manifestations of CEA are variable, even within a single litter and often the lesions in the two eyes are not similar in severity or distribution. One or more of the following signs can be observed in conjunction with CEA:

1. *Choroidal hypoplasia*. This is a lesion found temporal to the optic disc. It is an area with lack of pigment and tapetum, exposing sclera and abnormal choroidal vessels. The lesion is bilateral although the extent may vary between eyes. Choroidal hypoplasia in its mildest form may have little or no effect on vision, but major defects may cause some reduced vision due to absence of photo-

receptors and reduced numbers of ganglion cells and thinning of the nerve fiber layer of the retina [23]. Minor chorioretinal changes found on examination before three months of age can be masked by later pigmentation. Affected dogs, in which this phenomenon masks previous lesions are called 'go normals', and the condition is prevalent in a significant number of animals [24].

2. *Colobomas*. This defect is usually found at or in the vicinity of the optic disc. It is seen as a gray and/or white pit, either small and difficult to detect or larger with vessels dipping down over the rim. Small colobomas do not cause visual problems, but large ones, usually the size of the disc or more, may cause defective vision or blindness. Large colobomas involving the whole optic disc may predispose to retinal detachment.

3. *Retinal detachment*. The neural retina has partially or completely detached and can be observed floating in the vitreous. Detachment usually occur at an early age, before 7 weeks, but can occur also later in life, but usually before the age of 1 year. Vision is always severely affected with resultant blindness if complete and bilateral. Intraocular hemorrhage is common in conjunction with retinal detachment. Euthanasia is usually recommended in the most severe forms of CEA, i.e. dogs bilaterally blind because of large colobomas or retinal detachments.

Specific treatment

There is no effective treatment for CEA. It is important to induce preventive measures for the genetic defect. However, recommendations vary in different countries.

Early-onset photoreceptor dystrophies

The forms of progressive retinal atrophy (PRA) due to photoreceptor dysplasias have an early-onset. Table 5.3 summarises photoreceptor dysplasia or degeneration.

Rod–cone dysplasia (rcd)

Rod–cone dysplasia is an early onset retinal cell dystrophy characterized by a retarded differentiation of the rod and cone photoreceptors, followed by a subsequent degeneration. Affected breeds are the Irish Setter and the Collie. In the two dog breeds, the same biochemical abnormality is present; elevated retinal cGMP resulting from deficient retinal cGMP–PDE (cyclic guanosine monophosphate–phosphodiesterase) activity [25]. The defect has been shown to be inherited in a simple recessive mode, although the diseases are caused by genes at two different loci. The gene defect causal for rod cone dysplasia type one (red-1) in the Irish Setter has recently been identified [26, 27] and a DNA-based diagnostic test for the presence of the gene mutation has been developed [27, 28]. This test can be used to distinguish between dogs that are normal, heterozygous carriers, or homozygous affected at the rcd-1 gene locus [29]. In cats two specific families have been described having rod–cone dysplasia; a group of short-haired domestic cats in the USA and a strain of Abyssinian cats in England. In both the mode of inheritance for the defect had been shown to be dominant.

Clinical findings   These include initial night blindness followed by a progressive loss of day vision as well. Age of clinical signs is early, usually 6–12 weeks in dogs, somewhat earlier in cats (2–3 weeks). Blindness is apparent by 1–2 years in the dog and 12–16 weeks in the cat. Ophthalmoscopically the tapetal fundus is hyper-reflective, starting peripherally and spreading centrally. Within months there is a completely atrophic fundus with severe vascular attentuation. In the cat, nystagmus is often observed at an early age in affected animals. Early diagnosis of rod–cone dysplasia is performed by ERG, abnormalities being detectable at 4–6 weeks of age. In affected animals there are severely reduced or a lack of both rod and cone responses.

Rod dysplasia (rd)

This disease is characterized by a defective development of the rod photoreceptors with secondary degeneration of the cone system. The only breed in which the disease has been described so far is the Norwegian Elkhound [30].

Clinical findings   Initial night-blindness (nyctalopia) is detected in affected puppies at 2–3 months, while day vision is normal initially. Day and night vision deteriorate successively and affected dogs are blind at the age of 3–6 years. Ophthalmoscopically a granular and discolored appearance of the tapetal fundus is observed at 6–12 months progressing to tapetal hyper-reflectivity and vascular attenuation within a few years. Electroretinography at 6 weeks is diagnostic for the disease with a lack of rod responses and normal to slightly reduced cone responses in affected dogs.

Early retinal degeneration (erd)

Recently another recessively inherited retinal dystrophy has been described in the Norwegian Elkhound [31]. Morphologically there is an abnormal development of both rod and cone photoreceptors.

Clinical findings   Affected puppies are night blind at 6 weeks and completely blind at 1–1.5 years. Ophthalmoscopic signs of the dis-

Table 5.3 Some specific canine and feline inherited retinal diseases with primary photoreceptor involvement. The data summarizes information from the literature and the authors' personal experience

Breed	Disease/gene symbol	Mode of inherit.	Diagnosis by ophthalmoscopy	Diagnosis by ERG	ERG changes/responses
Irish Setter	rod–cone dysplasia type 1/rcd 1	AR	12–16 week (some have a later onset)	4–6 week	cone: ↓ rod: –
Collie	rod–cone dysplasia type 2/rcd 2	AR	12–16 week	4–6 week	cone: ↓ rod: –
Norwegian Elkhound	rod dysplasia/rd	AR	6 month	6 week	cone: N/↓ rod: –
Norwegian Elkhound	early retinal degeneration/erd	AR	6 month	6 week	a-wave domin., cone: ↓, rod: ↓
Miniature Schnauzer	photoreceptor dysplasia/pd	AR	2–5 yr	8 week	cone: N rod: ↓
Alaskan Malamute	cone degeneration (hemeralopia)	AR	4 yr (?)	6 week	cone: – rod: N
Miniature Longhaired Dachshund	progressive retinal atrophy	AR	5–7 month	4 month	cone: ↓ rod: ⇓
Papillon	progressive retinal degeneration	AR	13 month–2 yr	8 month	cone: ↓ rod: ⇓
Tibetan Spaniel	progressive retinal atrophy	AR	3–6 yr	≥1.5 yr	cone: ↓ rod: ⇓
Tibetan Terrier	progressive retinal atrophy	AR	1–1.5 yr	6–10 month	cone: ↓ rod: ⇓
Siberian Husky	X-linked progressive retinal degen./XL PRA	X-linked	1.5–2 yr	6–12 month	cone: ↓ rod: ⇓
Miniature Poodle	progressive rod cone degeneration/prcd	AR	3–5 yr	6–9 month	cone: ↓ rod: ⇓

Labrador Retriever	progressive rod cone degeneration/prcd	AR	2–6 yr	≥1.5 yr	cone: ↓ rod: ⇓
American Cocker Spaniel	progressive rod cone degeneration/prcd	AR	2–3 yr	1.5 yr	cone: ↓ rod: ⇓
English Cocker Spaniel	progressive rod cone degeneration/prcd	AR	3–6 yr	≥1.5 yr	cone: ↓ rod: ⇓
Abyssinian cat	rod cone dysplasia	AD	3 week	4–6 week	cone: − rod: −
Abyssinian cat	rod cone degeneration	AR	1.5–2 yr	8 month	cone: ↓ rod: ⇓

Symbols: AR, autosomal recessive; AD, autosomal dominant; N, normal; −, absent; ↓, decreased; ⇓, severely decreased.

ease may be observed at about 6 months and there is a retinal atrophy at the age of 1 year. Specifically the synaptic terminals are abnormal. ERG is diagnostic of the disease by 6 weeks of age; there is an a-wave dominated response which becomes non-recordable with age.

Photoreceptor dysplasia (pd)

A progressive retinal atrophy has recently been described in the Miniature Schnauzer dog and defined as a photoreceptor dysplasia [32]. The disease is characterized by unique morphologic and functional deficits during rod and cone development. The ophthalmoscopic diagnosis is only practicable very late in the disease process. Morphologically, however, changes are observed early in the photoreceptor outer segment layer as an area of short profiles of disorganized and disoriented disc membranes. The mode of inheritance for the gene defect is autosomal recessive.

Clinical findings   Retinal changes are not seen until 2–5 years of age by ophthalmoscopy. ERG can, however, provide evidence of disease by the age of 8 weeks. Affected puppies demonstrate significantly reduced dark-adapted b-wave response amplitudes to red or white light. There is no treatment for the defect except preventive measures taken through the breeding program.

Congenital retinal dystrophy

This is a hereditary and congenital disease of Briard dogs with a simple autosomal recessive inheritance [33]. Morphologic studies have shown changes in the retinal pigment epithelium with an accumulation of large vacuoles and inclusion bodies. It is not clear yet what the contents of these inclusions are but an accumulation of lipids are suspected. Ultrastructurally there is also disorganization of the rod photoreceptor outer segments at an early age but also with a successive involvement of the cone photoreceptors a few years later.

Clinical findings

Affected Briards are congenitally night blind but may have either normal or reduced daylight vision as well. Some affected dogs are both night- and day-blind. Ophthalmoscopically the fundus appears normal until the dogs are at least 3–4 years old. Then slight changes may be seen such as a subtle change in tapetal color and a slight vascular attenuation. The disease has extremely slow progression and deterioration of vision cannot be noticed clinically even through long-term studies (up to 7 years). Low amplitude or non-recordable rod responses are found with somewhat reduced cone responses by ERG, in affected puppies as young as 5-weeks of age.

Hemeralopia

Day blindness (hemeralopia) is an uncommon disease in the dog specifically described in the Alaskan Malamute [34]. The disease has an autosomal recessive inheritance. It is caused by a partial or total failure in development of cone photoreceptors.

Clinical findings

Clinical signs include day blindness but normal vision in darkness, often noticed at 2–6 months of age. ERG is diagnostic at an early age with abnormal cone responses and normal rod responses.

Malformation of the central nervous system resulting in blindness

This may include any disorder affecting the visual pathways. Detailed descriptions of these disorders are beyond the scope of this book, however, a brief survey of hydrocephalus is included.

Hydrocephalus

Hydrocephalus may be defined as a dilatation of the normally small, fluid-filled cavities and spaces (ventricles inside and subarachnoid space outside) of the brain with an increase in the volume of cerebrospinal fluid. In the dog, the most common form of hydrocephalus is congenital and with normal intracranial pressure in breeds with dome-shaped skulls. This condition often produces few clinical signs. The hydrocephalus may, however, become decompensated with increased intracranial pressure, causing ataxia and loss of higher functions such as vision, hearing, and intelligence. Involvement hydrocephalus in all breeds may develop secondarily to brain tumors, trauma, encephalitis, or meningitis.

An animal with hydrocephalus may present with few clinical signs obvious to the owner, as little cortical function is demanded of miniature breeds in many cases. Should, however, the disorder affect the visual cortex, visual impairment may result. Affection of the brainstem may compromise the optic nerve as well as the other cranial nerves necessary for normal eye function.

Clinical findings

The puppy may present only with the complaint of visual impairment. The pupils are dilated and direct and indirect pupillary light reflexes may be absent. The menace response is absent, but this may be difficult to evaluate even in normal puppies. A wandering nystagmus with rolling of the eyes in no specific pattern may be present. A thorough neurological examination usually reveals other neurological abnormalities as well. Open fontanelles and small skull bones are usually present, and the anterior part of the brain may protrude between the bones.

Diagnosis

A neurological examination will support the diagnosis, as well as the shape of the head and the breed of the affected animal. X-ray or other imaging techniques will establish the diagnosis.

Treatment and prognosis

Eventual treatment should be left to the neurologists. The prognosis for gaining vision in a congenitally blind animal is poor.

ACQUIRED VISUAL IMPAIRMENT – ACUTE ONSET

Acute visual impairment is an occurence which often makes both the patient and the owner distressed. Although the interest is easily focused only on the eyes, a detailed history should be taken and a thorough general physical examination of the patient should be performed, to rule out the presence of preceding or concurrent systemic disease and/or medication. It must also be remembered that even if the owner considers the visual impairment to be of sudden onset, the condition may have developed insidiously over a longer period of time.

Acute glaucoma

Acute glaucoma (see also Chapter 6) is in many ways the epitome of evil among eye diseases; it starts suddenly and unexpectedly, the course is accompanied by pain and the condition progresses irreversibly and promptly to blindness, if not treated. Different pathogenic mechanisms causing the high IOP in acute glaucoma produce similar clinical signs and a thorough examination is necessary to establish the cause of the condition.

Clinical signs

The pathologically elevated intraocular pressure (IOP) produces obvious clinical signs in dogs, whereas the clinical signs in cats are less prominent.

Signs of pain (e.g. blepharospasm, moderate epiphora, and altered behaviour), engorged episcleral vessels, corneal edema and a fixed, mid-sized pupil can be observed. The anterior chamber often appears shallower than normal, although this feature may be difficult to appreciate without experience. The cillary cleft usually appears closed when gonioscopy is performed. Retinal vessels are compressed, whereas changes in the optic nerve head are usually not detectable clinically in acute cases of glaucoma. The globe may be enlarged relatively early in the course of the disease, especially in young animals. The IOP is considerably elevated and tonometry readings of 50 to 70 mm Hg are common.

Diagnosis

The diagnosis of acute glaucoma is made on the basis of ocular signs. The presence of an elevation of the IOP is the most important clinical sign. The firmness of the globe caused by the high IOP can usually be palpated, but palpation is a very rough and sometimes unreliable method to estimate the IOP. Measuring the IOP with a tonometer is therefore strongly recommended to obtain an initial IOP value and to verify the diagnosis (pp. 18–20 and 21). Gonioscopy should always be performed to evaluate the appearance of the iridocorneal angle (p. 22). Corneal edema makes the gonioscopic view obscure and in patients with unilateral glaucoma gonioscopy should also be performed on the normotensive eye to get hints of the cause of the glaucoma.

Differential diagnosis

Acute conjunctivitis causes the eye to look red, but in conjunctivitis the conjunctiva is pink or reddish and the individual vessels are not prominent. Furthermore, the conjunctival vessels are easily moveable, unlike the episcleral ones. Orbital disease or episcleritis may cause episcleral injection but intraocular disease is not usually present. Orbital disease may cause pupillary abnormalities and uveitis may occur with episcleritis.

Corneal edema is seen in several other diseases (e.g. ulcerative keratitis, endothelial dystrophy, and uveitis), but neither dilation of the pupil nor elevation of the IOP is present in these diseases.

Iris atrophy causes the pupil to look dilated. Dilated pupils, unresponsive to light stimulus, can be seen in several other diseases, including advanced stages of retinal degeneration and optic neuritis. Retinal degeneration also causes attenuation of retinal vessels, which look similar to the vessel compression in acute glaucoma.

In rare patients with primary open-angle glaucoma, the IOP is slightly elevated for a long period of time, sometimes years, causing very subtle signs which are often neglected by the owner. In advanced stages of this form of glaucoma, the ciliary cleft is likely to collapse, which causes a sudden, severe increase in the IOP mimicking acute glaucoma. The possibility of an insidious, chronic glaucoma preceding the acute, severe elevation in IOP should be considered in patients where signs of an acute glaucoma and unexpected findings indicative of chronic glaucoma are seen simultaneously.

Treatment and prognosis

(Further details of treatment can be found on pp. 186–188). Acute glaucoma is an emergency. The treatment should aim at retrieving vision, but in cases where vision is already lost, the aim is to keep the animal comfortable and without pain.

Medical treatment should be initiated immediately to lower the IOP to a physiological level. If the glaucoma is secondary to another disease, the primary cause has to be treated as well. Repeated tonometry is essential to evaluate the response to the therapy. If IOP is not lowered sufficiently or returns to pathological levels, surgical treatment is necessary. The animal should not leave the clinic before the IOP is controlled. A combination of medical and surgical treatments is often required for long-term success. In patients with unilateral primary glaucoma, it is important to treat the unaffected eye prophylactically [35] and to inform the owner of the bilateral potential of the disease.

Correct diagnosis and successful lowering of the IOP very early in the course of the condition are essential for a favorable outcome. Highly elevated IOP (greater than 50 mm Hg) may cause severely impaired vision within less than 1 day, whereas an IOP of 40 mm Hg usually results in blindness within 3 to 4 days.

Intraocular hemorrhage

Intraocular hemorrhage can be caused by several different pathogenic mechanisms. The extent of blood within the eye, as well as the location of the hemorrhage, may vary considerably. Several conditions causing neovascularization and/or the leakage of blood from intraocular vessels can be listed:

- Hemorrhage in the anterior chamber
    trauma
    pre-iridal fibrovascular membranes
    anterior uveitis
    intraocular neoplasia
    coagulation factor disorders or platelet disorders
    retinal detachment
    PHTVL/PHPV
- Hemorrhage in the lens or in a retrolental plaque
    PHTVL/PHPV

- Hemorrhage in the vitreous cavity or in the retina
    chorioretinitis
    coagulation factor disorders or platelet disorders
    systemic lupus erythematosus
    hyperviscosity syndrome
    diabetes mellitus
    hypertensive retinopathy
    retinal detachment
    PHTVL/PHPV

Clinical signs

Hemorrhage in the anterior chamber, hyphema, is easily detectable (Figure 5.9). In complete hyphema, the blood turns bluish-black after approximately 1 week. This is often referred to as eight-ball hyphema (from the color of ball number 8 in pool). Hemorrhage in the posterior part of the eye may often require use of a slit-lamp or ophthalmoscope to be visualized. The location of hemorrhage within the retina can be established ophthalmoscopically by shape and color. Furthermore, it is valuable to establish whether the blood is clotted or not. Clotted blood in the anterior chamber is often seen when the cause is anterior uveitis or trauma, whereas hemorrhage caused by coagulation disorders is unclotted.

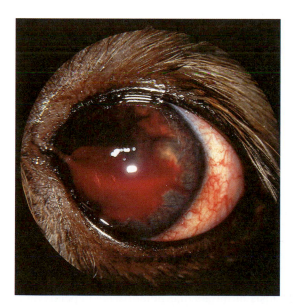

Figure 5.9   Blunt trauma to the eye of this dog caused hyphema, traumatic uveitis, and the development of iris bombé.

Diagnosis

The owners should be asked if the pet may have eaten toxic substances, e.g. rodenticides containing anticoagulants, or if abnormal bleeding has been noticed previously. Recurrent hemorrhages are often indicative of a neoplastic or congenital origin. Breed disposition, for example, CEA in collies and PHTVL/PHPV in Dobermann Pinschers, concurrent systemic diseases, for example, feline viral leukaemia and immune-mediated thrombocytopenia, and the age of the patient (congenital diseases) should be considered.

A general clinical examination including the testing of hematological parameters should always be performed. Coagulation screening can be used to rule out coagulopathies. Examination of littermates may give clues to the cause when excessive hemorrhage is found in young animals. Intraocular pressure should be measured, because excessive hemorrhage in the anterior chamber may impair aqueous drainage and cause secondary glaucoma. Ultrasonography may be useful to detect intraocular neoplasms, vitreal hemorrhage, and retinal detachment in blood-filled eyes.

Treatment and prognosis

It is not possible to lay out general rules for treatment of intraocular hemorrhage. However, some suggestions on treatment of hyphema are:

● Treatment of concurrent uveitis is essential in hyphema to avoid inflammatory sequelae. It should be noted that non-steroidal anti-inflammatory drugs should be used cautiously, because these drugs interfere with thrombocytic function. Furthermore, mydriatics should be used with caution in excessive hyphema; mydriatics may contribute to impairment of aqueous humor outflow in these cases. IOP should be monitored when mydriatics are used. If a secondary glaucoma is elicited, mydriatics should be discontinued immediately and medical treatment to lower the IOP should be started.
● In patients with excessive hyphema and elevated IOP, removal of blood elements by irrigation of the anterior chamber may be advantageous. Intracameral injection or addition of fibrinolytic agents [36] to the irrigation solution will lyse clots and enhance their physiologic removal. Surgical removal of large clots may occasionally be performed.

The prognosis of intraocular hemorrhage depends on the cause and the extent of the intraocular lesions. It is often advisable not to give a prognosis until resorption of the blood allows inspection of the intraocular structures in cases where severe hemorrhage obscures the view. Additional information is given in other sections of this book concerning diseases which cause intraocular hemorrhage.

SARD

SARD (sudden acquired retinal degeneration) is a retinal degenerative disease which occurs acutely in adult dogs. The cause of the disease is still unknown [37]. Although the fundus appearance in affected animals is normal (Figure 5.10) there are marked morphological changes. A rapid loss of photoreceptor outer segments is seen by ultrastructure (Figure 5.11) followed by degeneration of the other retinal layers. No breed is particularly susceptible and crossbreeds have also been affected by the disease. Most often, the affected animal is of middle-age and appears to be in good general health. In some instances there has been a history of polyphagia, polyuria, polydipsia, together with elevations in the levels of serum alkaline phosphatase (SAP), serum alanine amino transferase (SAAT), serum cholesterol, or serum bilirubin. It has been speculated that these changes may be symptoms of the physiologic stress associated with the unidentified retinotoxic factor.

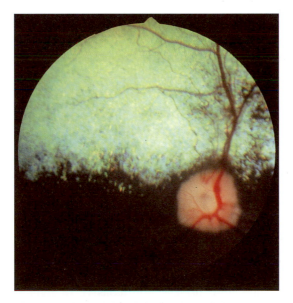

Figure 5.10 The fundus appearance is normal in this acutely blind (for about 4 weeks) 4 year old Dachshund with sudden acquired retinal degeneration (SARD).

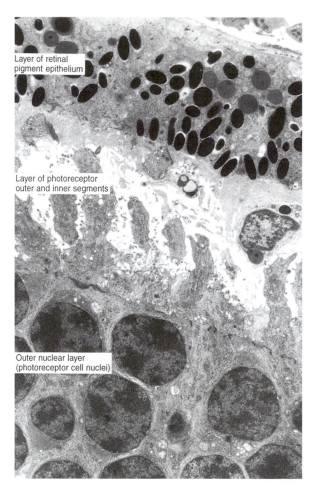

Layer of retinal
pigment epithelium

Layer of photoreceptor
outer and inner segments

Outer nuclear layer
(photoreceptor cell nuclei)

Figure 5.11   Electron micrograph of the outer retina of the case in Figure 5.10. Obvious degenerative changes are observed in the photoreceptor outer and inner segment layer. Initial magnification: × 2600 (now × 2080).

Clinical findings

Affected dogs lose their vision completely and irreversibly within 1–2 weeks. Clinical examination shows moderately to widely dilated pupils, which are more or less unresponsive to light stimuli. The fundus appearance is normal, but the ERG is non-recordable. After several weeks or months there is ophthalmoscopic evidence of a generalized retinal degeneration.

Differential diagnosis

SARD can be differentiated from optic neuritis by the totally extinguished ERG. It might in the late stage of the disease be more difficult to differentiate SARD from generalized retinal degeneration from other causes, such as hereditary rod–cone degeneration, in which the ERG is also non-recordable. Another differential diagnosis is CNS neoplasia, in which sudden-onset blindness may occur. However the ERG is not often extinguished in such cases.

Treatment

There is no effective treatment for SARD.

Retinal detachment

Retinal detachment is a rather common finding in the small animal ophthalmic practice. It is usually the result of a separation of the neural retina from the retinal pigment epithelium through maldevelopment (as in CEA or RD), vitreal traction, exudation or transudation (as in chorioretinitis and hypertension), or associated with retinal tears or holes that may occur with a hereditary predisposition in brachycephalic breeds, as a sequelae to trauma or atrophy or as a complication of cataract or lens luxation surgery. Detachments due to

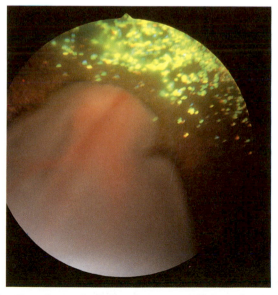

Figure 5.12 Complete retinal detachment and disinsersion in a 2 year old Tibetan Terrier. The hyper-reflective and avascular fundus (without neural retina) might be confused with complete retinal atrophy.

tears or holes are referred to as rhegmatogenous. In severe cases the neural retina may be separated over its whole area, only remaining attached at the optic disc and at the *ora ciliaris retinae*. When the latter attachment is completely separated, a veil of retinal tissue may hang loosely down from the optic disc (Figure 5.12). Separation of the photoreceptors from the choriocapillaris and retinal pigment epithelium causes photoreceptor degeneration.

Clinical findings

Acute-onset of severe visual impairment or blindness is a common sequelae to retinal detachment. In partial detachments there are usually no obvious clinical signs due to the detachment. Pupillary light reflexes are abnormal to normal depending on extent and duration of the lesion. Ophthalmoscopically, a grayish veil-like structure is seen floating in the vitreous, with clearly visible retinal vessels. If the retina is only partly detached, areas become elevated as flat or bullous regions that are out of focus compared to normal areas and the optic disc. There may be accompanying signs of systemic disease (Figure 5.13).

Differential diagnosis

An important differential diagnosis in retinal detachment is end-stage retinal atrophy. When the retina is completely detached and not

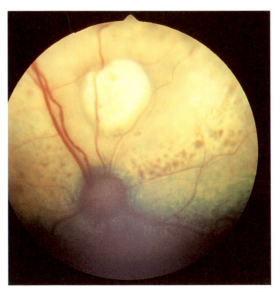

Figure 5.13   Partial retinal detachment with a neuroretinal hole and elevation of large areas of the neural retina in conjunction with hypertension in a 12 year old Persian cat.

fastened at the *ora ciliaris retinae*, the neural tissue may not always be easily seen by the examiner, who might only observe the hyper-reflective tapetal fundus without retinal vessels (Figure 5.12).

Treatment and prognosis

Treatment of early cases and especially partial retinal detachment is sometimes possible depending on etiology. Chorioretinitis cases have the most favorable prognosis where treatment consists of anti-inflammatory medication as well as treatment directed towards the primary cause. Mild to moderate serous detachments often respond to a combination of a diuretics and systemic corticosteroids. The surgical treatment of rhegmatogenous retinal detachments is attempted less frequently in small animals compared to humans because most cases in animals are not diagnosed early enough. Methods of surgical treatment include cryopexy of holes and tears, drainage of subretinal fluid, application of scleral buckle, and filling the posterior segment with air, gas, or silicone oil. Prognosis for large and complete detachments is poor.

Hypertensive retinopathy

Hypertensive retinopathy is not an uncommon disease in small animal practice and occurs most often in older cats. In addition to acute blindness or severe visual impairment, affected animals usually have an elevated systolic arterial blood pressure (often greater than 200 mm Hg), elevated blood urea nitrogen and creatinine levels, and in some cases cardiac abnormalities as well. It is often difficult to evaluate which disease process comes first; a primary renal disease, which may cause hypertension or primary hypertension causing secondary cardiac and renal abnormalities (Figure 5.14). Hyperthyroidism is a common potential cause in older cats.

Clinical findings

The typical presenting complaint is acute vision loss. Ophthalmoscopically there are often bilateral severe retinal changes, such as retinal and vitreal hemorrhage, elevation or detachment of all or parts of the neural retina, and retinal vascular tortuosity.

Treatment and prognosis

Therapy is directed towards treatment of the primary disease. Hypotensive therapy is initiated and, in some cases, diuretics. Therapy is usually somewhat effective regarding the elevated blood pressure. Early treatment of less severe retinal lesions gives return of vision in some cases although the long-term prognosis is poor. Most cases of

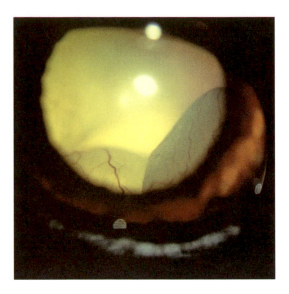

Figure 5.14 Bullous retinal detachment seen through the pupil in a 10 year old Border Collie with primary renal disease and hypertension.

hypertensive retinopathy are advanced, however, with little or no effect of treatment.

Optic neuritis

Optic neuritis is an inflammation of the optic nerve, either at the level of the globe or closer to the brain. The potential causes include specific infections, such as toxoplasmosis, extension of inflammation from adjacent tissues, neoplasia, the influence of toxins, and trauma. Immune-mediated causes are often suspected although the majority of such cases are categorized as idiopathic.

Clinical findings

Affected animals are often presented with bilateral acute-onset blindness. The pupils are widely dilated and the pupillary light reflexes are lost. Ophthalmoscopically the disc may appear swollen and indistinct and sometimes small hemorrhages are observed at or in the vicinity of the disc (Figure 5.15). The adjacent retina may also be affected. The ERG is usually only somewhat reduced or may be normal. In some cases of optic neuritis, with inflammatory lesions closer to the brain, the fundus appears normal.

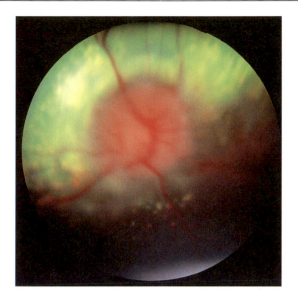

Figure 5.15   Optic neuritis in a 4 year old Bichon Frisé with acute-onset blindness.

Differential diagnosis

SARD is an important differential in optic neuritis, although in SARD the ERG is non-recordable and PLRs usually present but sluggish. Central blindness is another differential. In such cases pupillary reflexes are often normal, the animal has other CNS symptoms and the fundus and optic disc are often normal appearing. Reticulosis (see below) is another differential. In papilledema, there is a non-inflammatory swelling of the optic disc, usually associated with compression of the retrobulbar part of the optic nerve by tumor or associated with systemic hypertension. Vision is not impaired in papilledema and pupillary light reflexes and ERG are normal.

Treatment and prognosis

Optic neuritis is treated by systemic corticosteroids in high doses initially (2–3 weeks) then, as long-term treatment at lower levels, every other day up to several months. The underlying cause should be treated if possible. In specific infections, broad spectrum antibiotics are indicated. The prognosis is guarded with recurrence of the disease being a common sequelae.

Central blindness

Central blindness or amaurosis describes visual impairment with normal ocular findings, in which the lesion can be localized to the visual pathway within the brain [1, 2]. Often signs other than visual disturbances will be present. Apparent blindness is, however, often the first sign noted by the owner. In managing a neurologic problem, the first step is localization of the disease process to a single anatomic site. This may be useful, for example when neoplasia is suspected. The disorders may be focal and affecting only one part of the CNS system. Lesions involving most of the CNS are categorized as multi-focal, systemic, or diffuse. Some of them may initially appear as focal diseases but progress to affect other structures. Examples of systemic or multifocal signs involving the visual pathway are brain stem lesions involving cranial nerves and cerebral lesions affecting the visual cortex. The major disease categories producing multifocal signs are degenerative, metabolic, neoplastic, nutritional, inflammatory, and toxic disorders.

Reticulosis

This is a malignant inflammatory condition seen in the dog, but rarely in the cat. The condition is considered either inflammatory or neoplastic by various authors. Reticulosis has a prevelence for white matter and may infiltrate the optic nerves causing diffuse or focal lesions, including atrophy or swelling of the optic disc, depending on the degree of involvement. White matter of the brainstem, cerebellum, and upper cervical spinal cord may also be affected. The disease may affect dogs of all ages.

Clinical findings

Acute or gradual vision loss in one or both eyes is the main clinical sign when the optic nerves are affected. The condition does not seem to cause pain, unless the upper cervical spinal cord is involved. Lesions in this area will produce neck stiffness. In the ocular form of reticulosis, the pupil is dilated and the menace reaction as well as direct and consensual pupillary light reflexes are absent on the affected side. ERG shows a normal retinal function unless the nerve fiber layer of the retina is involved.

Differential diagnosis

The most important diagnosis is optic neuritis, which clinically will be indistinguishable from reticulosis of the optic nerve. In fact, reticulosis may be considered one form of optic neuritis. However, not all cases of optic neuritis are reticulosis.

Sudden acquired retinal degeneration (SARD) also causes acute vision loss. ERG is non-recordable. SARD will not improve on corticosteroid therapy, in contrast to reticulosis.

Treatment and prognosis

The disease responds to treatment with corticosteroids, but long-term treatment with high doses of steroids or other immune suppressive agents may be necessary. Recurrence of signs usually occurs when steroid doses are reduced below therapeutic levels. Thus, the prognosis is considered guarded.

Encephalitis

Inflammation of the brain tissue is referred to as encephalitis and inflammation of the meninges covering the brain as meningitis. When both occur simultaneously, the disease is called a meningoencephalitis. The condition is caused by several infectious agents, both viral and bacterial. In cats, the most important is feline infectious peritonitis (FIP), usually of the dry form, causing granulomatous inflammation in the CNS. Ocular signs, notably intraocular inflammation (uveitis often with keratitic precipitates in cats), may accompany the CNS findings. In dogs distemper must be included in the differential diagnosis of any dog with neurologic signs. Accompanying ocular signs may include conjunctivitis, KCS, optic neuritis and retinitis, as well as Horner's syndrome (ptosis, miosis, enophthalmos, and protrusion of the third eyelid) due to lesions of the sympathetic innervation.

Clinical findings

Depending on the site of the lesion within the brain, neurologic signs will be variable. There is usually evidence of more than one focus (multifocal) of CNS damage. In lesions involving the visual cortex, central blindness may develop. If the lower parts of the visual pathway are intact, clinical findings may include lack of menace responses, but with pupillary light reflexes present. Signs develop over a few days in most infections, but in FIP onset may be insidious. There is often a slight elevation of body temperature.

Differential diagnosis

Any other multifocal brain disease may produce similar signs. Examination of cerebrospinal fluid as well as blood chemistry and serology are important factors in establishing a diagnosis.

Treatment

Broad-spectrum antibiotics should be used when a bacterial infection is suspected. A normal blood–brain barrier may be difficult to penetrate for many antibiotics, however, when an infection is present, the barrier is broken down, permitting penetrance of several antibacterial agents. Symptomatic supportive treatment will also be necessary.

Intoxications

CNS signs can result from endogenous (produced within the body) toxins as well as exogenous (ingested, inhaled, absorbed through the skin) toxins. Hepatic encephalopathy is described later as an effect of an endogenous toxin.

A history of exposure to a toxic agent is the most important factor establishing the diagnosis in cases of exogenous poisoning. Therefore, the owner must be questioned carefully in an attempt to find a possible source. CNS signs other than central blindness will often be more obvious in exogenous intoxications. For identification of toxic agents, treatment and prognosis, the reader is referred to textbooks on this topic.

ACQUIRED VISUAL IMPAIRMENT – CHRONIC PROGRESSIVE ONSET

A chronic progressive onset of visual impairment is often difficult to detect by the owner. It is not uncommon that blinding disorders of this type are elucidated by chance in conjunction with examination or treatment of an animal for other causes than ophthalmic problems. Several disease processes of this type are, furthermore, either breed-related and in many cases hereditary. Through schemes in the various countries for eradication of hereditary eye diseases, many potential blinding disorders of chronic progressive onset are discovered.

Phthisis bulbus

Phthisis bulbus, a degenerated, shrunken eye, can develop secondary to severe damage to the ciliary body with decreased aqueous humor production and resultant hypotension. There is commonly a history of severe ocular trauma or chronic uveitis. The condition develops over a long period of time, usually months, and the end stage is a globe of considerably less size than normal with disorganized contents (Figure 5.16).

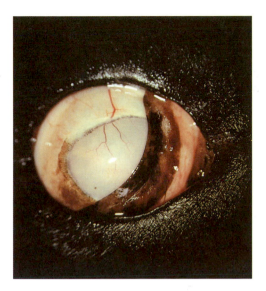

Figure 5.16 A middle-aged English Springer Spaniel with phthisis bulbus of the right eye.

Clinical signs

The globe is considerably smaller than normal and the cornea is opaque and vascularization with pigmentation present in variable degrees. Phthisis bulbus is usually unilateral and the size of the globe diminishes gradually over months. Signs of intraocular inflammation may be noted when the cornea is still transparent. Vision is lost when the globe has become phthisical.

Differential diagnosis

Microphthalmos is a differential diagnosis to phthisis bulbus. Microphthalmus is a congenital condition which develops without preceding ocular trauma or intraocular inflammation. Enophthalmos may mimic microphthalmos in appearance; the globe will be relatively normal.

Treatment

Chronic intraocular inflammation may cause discomfort. The relationship between the eyelids and the globe is disturbed and recurrent conjunctivitis is a common problem. Furthermore, the cosmesis of a phthisical globe is usually poor. Enucleation is often the best solution for the animal, but in patients where the globe is maintained, palliative treatment of conjunctivitis with irrigation and topical medications is necessary. A relationship between primary ocular sarcomas and concurrent chronic uveitis, which may cause phthisis bulbi, has been suggested in cats [38]. Thus, enucleation is probably to be recommended in this species.

Corneal disease

The transparency of the cornea is necessary for normal vision. This transparency is due to the cornea's state of relative dehydration, avascularity, lack of pigmentation, and the regular arrangement of stromal collagen fibrils. In order for the cornea to remain healthy, the eyelids must be normal in shape and functional, the tear film must be normal, and there must not be any inflammatory processes present in the cornea. In chronic corneal diseases, the cornea gradually changes appearance. This may be caused by edema, neovascularization, granulation tissue formation, scarring, and pigmentation. A thorough description of corneal diseases is given in Chapter 4; however, chronic diseases leading to visual impairment are briefly mentioned here. These include keratoconjunctivitis sicca, pigmentary keratitis, chronic superficial keratitis, punctate keratitis, corneal dystrophies, and endothelial dystrophy.

Keratoconjunctivitis sicca (KCS) (see pp. 218–222)

The condition is caused by a tear deficiency, most often because of an inflammatory reaction of the lacrimal gland [39]. Acute tear deficiency may cause corneal ulceration and perforation. More common, however, is a chronic disease with progressive deterioration in vision due to corneal changes.

Clinical findings

Typically, there is a history of chronic conjunctivitis with an accumulation of tenacious mucus on and around the eye. Conjunctivitis and keratitis evolve when the ocular surface dries and desiccates. Abnormal hypertrophy of the inflamed conjunctiva causes redundant pleating folds. Opportunistic bacteria can be cultured from the ocular discharge, but their abundance is secondary to the effect of KCS. Corneal changes include vascularization, scarring, and pigmentation and may progress to involve the whole cornea. If the cornea has normal sensory innervation, this leads to marked discomfort. However, the corneal nerves are usually damaged and insensitive in canine KCS, thus the condition is not associated with severe pain. A Schirmer tear test will reveal subnormal values. Treatment is discussed in Chapter 7, but usually includes daily cleaning, tear replacement therapy and/or topical instillation of cyclosporine.

Pigmentary keratitis

This condition is a corneal response to chronic irritation. Exophthalmic breeds are most susceptible and several factors can be responsible for the pigmentation:

- KCS – even moderately lowered tear production may produce clinical signs, as a large portion of the globe is exposed in brachyocephalic dogs.
- Lagophthalmos – the animal is not able to close the eyelids completely. On close questioning, an owner may state that the animal sleeps with the eyelids only partly closed. A reduced blinking frequency with poor distribution of the tears may also be present.
- Trichiasis – hairs from the area adjacent to the eye rub on the cornea.

Treatment

Treatment of pigmentary keratitis includes removal of the initiating cause, such as canthoplasty. Medical treatment may include frequent topical application of tear substituting eye drops, topical cyclosporine, and in some cases also corticosteroids, depending on the cause of the condition.

Chronic superficial keratitis (CSK)

Several names have been used for this disease, such as Überreiter's disease, keratitis pigmentosa, and pannus. The main cause appears to be an immunologic reaction, with exposure to sunlight triggering the disease and aggravating the clinical signs [40]. The disease may occasionally be seen in dogs of any breed, but the majority of cases are diagnosed in the German Shepherd and related breeds [41]. A genetic predisposition is considered likely. The condition occurs bilaterally in middle-aged dogs, with males and females equally affected. A chronic inflammation of the nictitating membrane, called plasmacytic conjunctivitis, is often also prevalent in dogs affected with CSK.

Clinical signs

Corneal changes include cellular infiltration, extensive vascularization and formation of granulation tissue which may be heavily pigmented. Initial changes are often seen in the ventrolateral parts of the cornea, in untreated cases progressing to involve the whole cornea. Schirmer tear test values are normal or elevated because of irritation. The surface of the nictitating membrane, especially near the rim, may have a coblestone-like appearance.

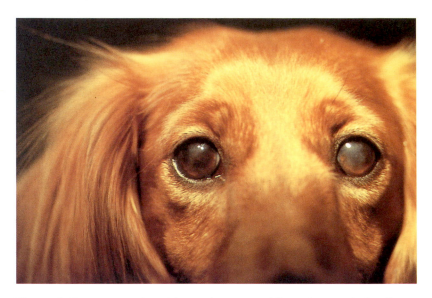

Figure 5.17 Punctate keratitis causing severe bilateral corneal cloudiness and partial pigmentation in a 6 year old long-haired Dachshund

Treatment

Treatment is lifelong and consists mainly of topical application of corticosteroids and/or cyclosporine. The results of treatment may be remarkably successful, but the condition will recur if treatment is discontinued.

Superficial punctate keratitis

The term describes a diffuse, ulcerative keratitis that is recurrent, bilateral and symmetric (Figure 5.17) [42]. The condition affects mainly the long-haired Dachshund, but sporadically dogs of other breeds may also be affected. The disease is considered to be immune-mediated, although the pathogenesis is not completely understood.

Clinical findings

The condition may be acute and painful with bilateral epiphora and blepharospasm. More chronic onset, however, is not uncommon. A number of small gray spots that may be fluorescein positive in the initial stage are seen in the cornea, and some edema may be present. After some days, neovascularization as an attempt at healing of the cornea develops. As the condition becomes chronic, a combination of punctate ulcers, vascularization, and pigmentation can be observed. The changes gradually progress to involve the whole cornea. Acute episodes with pain and deeper ulcers may occur and occasional descemetoceles and melting ulcers may aggravate the situation.

Treatment and prognosis

Treatment is lifelong and consists mainly of corticosteroids and/or cyclosporine topically plus antibiotics topically in secondary bacterial infection. Deep or perforated ulcers may demand surgical treatment.

Corneal lipid dystrophy and degeneration (see pp. 72–73)

Corneal stromal dystrophy is a non-inflammatory, most often bilateral condition, which may be caused by accumulation of lipid within the cornea [43]. The term dystrophy is usually reserved for the forms thought to have inherited basis. The deposits most commonly occur in the central parts of the cornea, in the outer stromal layers. The epithelium is not usually involved in the dystrophy. Vision is not usually affected, but in certain cases the whole cornea may be involved. *Arcus lipoides corneae*, where the lipid is located in the periphery, occurs more rarely.

Clinical findings

The dystrophic area may present as a shiny, fairly well demarcated zone in the middle area of the cornea. Lipid crystals may resemble tiny needles, but in degenerations and lipid keratopathies may be denser and break through the corneal epithelium. If the epithelium is intact, the condition is not painful.

Treatment

If secondary to other disease, this should be identified and treated. Accumulations in the stroma not impairing vision do not require treatment.

Corneal edema and endothelial dysfunction

Corneal edema in the absence of other findings may be due to a dysfunction of the endothelial cells [44]. The corneal endothelium is a single cell layer and, if injured, the cells have little regenerative capacity. To compensate, they will stretch to cover a large area. This has been described as a familiar disorder (endothelial dystrophy) in the Boston Terrier (Figure 5.18) and probably in the Airedale Terrier, and is seen sporadically in older dogs of all breeds.

Corneal edema may also result from other ocular diseases, such as glaucoma, uveitis, and ulcerative keratitis. A hazy cornea mimicking corneal edema occurs in mucopolysaccharidosis IV, a metabolic disorder in the cat.

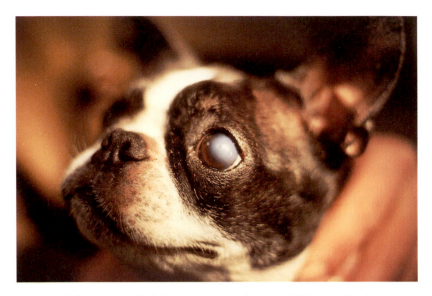

Figure 5.18   Endothelial dystrophy in an 8 year old Boston Terrier.

Clinical findings

The edematous cornea is opaque, complicating examination of the inner structures of the eye. The cornea is gray to light blue with a spongy appearance. If not associated with other painful ocular diseases, the condition is painless. There is usually an absence scleral injection, and the cornea is fluorescein negative. Bullous keratopathy may complicate the disease in advanced stages and cause painful and persistent ulceration. If bilateral, vision may be impaired.

Treatment and prognosis

If secondary to another eye disease, the primary disease must be diagnosed and treated properly. Topical osmotic agents have been tried to desiccate the cornea, but with little effect. Thermal keratoplasty or the placement of permant thin conjuctival flaps may be of value. Full thickness corneal transplanation may restore vision, but rejection of donor tissue may occur. The prognosis for restoration of vision must therefore be considered guarded.

Chronic uveitis and its sequelae

Uveitis is an inflammation of the vascular tunics of the eye, which can be subdivided into iritis, cyclitis, and choroiditis depending on the part of the uvea which is affected. Anterior uveitis or iridocyclitis refers to an inflammation of both the iris and the ciliary body.

Multiple etiologies are capable of causing uveitis in cats and dogs (see Chapter 6). Chronic uveitis is a potential threat to both vision and eye. Cats are more commonly presented with the condition than dogs.

Aspects of the pathogenesis

The pathogenesis of chronic and recurrent uveitis is still poorly understood, but immunologic reactions are involved. Alterations of the vascular structure and/or permeability of uveal blood vessels may persist after the acute stages of an extensive, uncontrolled inflammation. A subsequent tendency for circulating immune complexes to be deposited in vessels with increased permeability has been reported. Furthermore, the property of the vitreous body in acting as a reservoir for antigens and persisting sensitized lymphocytes may be of importance.

Clinical signs

The condition may be uni- or bilateral. Bilateral involvement is commonly seen in patients with infectious or autoimmune diseases, whereas unilateral chronic uveitis may initially be caused by severe trauma to the eye or unilateral lens disease.

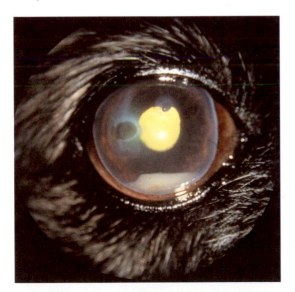

Figure 5.19 Acute uveitis as a result of a corneal foreign body of 1 weeks duration in a 3 year old Pekinese. Except for the corneal defect there is corneal edema, hypopyon, small and irregular pupil, and obvious swelling of the iris. The intraocular pressure is lowered.

The clinical signs of acute uveitis include pain and discomfort, ciliary flush, miosis, aqueous flare and cell, precipitates of cells on fibrin on the corneal endothelial surface and anterior lens capsule, spongy swollen iris, and lowered IOP (Figure 5.19), but will vary dependent upon intensity, distribution, (anterior vs. posterior segment) and duration of the inflammation. Additional clinical signs in chronic uveitis may include:

- Neovascularization of the iris with or without engorgement of the iris vessels. Preiridal fibrovascular membranes or *rubeosis iridis* can be observed as randomly organized vessels compared to the normal iris vessels which are arranged in a radial fashion. The neovascularization is usually more prominent in cats compared to dogs.
- Changes in iris pigmentation. The iris is usually diffusely hyper-pigmented in the affected eye. Dispersed pigment may be observed on the anterior lens capsule. Iridal lymphocytic nodules appearing as circular reddish-brown to grey lesions with a diameter of 1–2 mm are not uncommon in chronic uveitis in cats.
- Secondary iris atrophy.
- Various sequelae including corneal changes, intraocular adhesions (synechiae), intraocular membranes, secondary cataracts, secondary retinal diseases, or glaucoma may be present.
- Partial visual impairment or blindness.

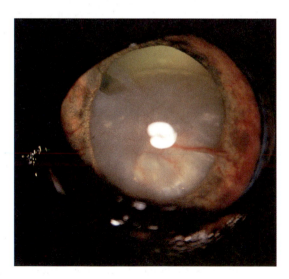

Figure 5.20   Sequelae of chronic uveitis in a 13 year old cat: fibrovascular membranes, cataracts, and lens luxation.

Sequelae

A number of vision threatening conditions may be caused by uveitis (Figure 5.20). Thus, early diagnosis and proper treatment of the initial inflammation is essential to prevent or reduce the development of potentially harmful sequelae.

Corneal changes. Uveitis may interfere with the water-pumping ability of the corneal endothelium causing corneal edema. Furthermore, keratitis with pigmentation and vascularization is not uncommon.

Intraocular adhesions form when the inflamed iris sticks to other structures in the eye. The initial fibrinous adhesions are followed by fibrovascular organization. Adhesions between iris and cornea peripherally (peripheral anterior synechiae) may impair aqueous outflow. Posterior synechiae, adhesions between iris and lens, are commonly seen at the edge of the pupil. Posterior synechiae affecting only parts of the circumference of the pupil may cause distortion of the pupil. If the posterior synechiae affects the entire circumference of the pupil (*seclusio pupillae*) aqueous humor is trapped in the posterior segment of the eye. This implies that the IOP will be higher in the posterior segment than in the anterior chamber, which results in forward ballooning of the iris, or iris bombé (Figure 5.9). Exudates or blood in the pupil may cause formation of tissue membranes across the pupil (from iris to iris). Membranes covering the entire pupil will cause an occlusion of the pupil. High aqueous protein levels, for example due to protein exudation or intraocular hemorrhage are considered to predispose for synechiae formation.

Cyclitic membranes are fibrovascular membranes extending from the ciliary body across the pupil and/or across the anterior face of the vitreous body.

Secondary cataracts may form, probably as a result of alterations in the aqueous humor.

Lens luxation may occur in eyes with chronic uveitis. Decrease in strength and subsequent rupture of the lens zonules have been proposed to be a sequelae to intraocular inflammation, especially in cats.

Secondary glaucoma may arise from several different mechanisms in conjunction with uveitis. Impaired aqueous flow because of inflammation and deposition of inflammatory cells debris in the outflow pathways, peripheral anterior synechia, and seclusion or occlusion of the pupil may cause elevation of IOP.

Secondary retinal degeneration may be caused by extension of choroiditis to involve both the choroid and the retina (chorioretinitis) or inflammatory effects on the choriocapillaris and/or RPE.

Exudative retinal detachment may be seen in patients with choroiditis, where the retina is elevated by subretinal fluid, or secondary to traction of intravitreal or cyclitic membranes caused by intraocular inflammation or hemorrhage.

Phthisis bulbus. Chronic uveitis may cause severe ciliary body atrophy which implies decreased aqueous humor formation and pathologically lowered IOP.

Diagnosis

The diagnosis is based on history and clinical findings. General physical examination, blood biochemistry, hematology, and serology may be of value, although the etiology is frequently difficult to establish. It must be remembered that the uveitis may have developed secondarily to some other primary ocular disease.

Aqueous, vitreous or subretinal paracentesis may be indicated for cytology and microbial isolation. Results are often unspecific and the procedure may even cause exacerbation of the inflammation. However, results of diagnostic value are most likely to be found in eyes with visible exudates or in lymphosarcoma suspects [45]. The risk of hemorrhage must be considered before vitreous paracentesis is performed.

Differential diagnosis

Conjunctivitis causes the eye to look red, but in conjunctivitis the conjunctiva is pink or reddish and the underlying individual episcleral vessels are not prominent. Furthermore, the conjunctival vessels are easily moved, on the contrary to the straight perilimbal anterior ciliary vessels, which cause the ciliary flush seen in uveitis.

Corneal edema is seen in several other diseases, such as ulcerative keratitis, endothelial dystrophy, and glaucoma. In chronic anterior uveitis, however, there are other signs of chronic inflammatory disease.

Primary iris atrophy can be distinguished from iris atrophy secondary to chronic uveitis by the presence of other clinical signs of intraocular inflammation in the latter condition.

Cataracts may cause secondary lens-induced uveitis. The history, breed, and age of the patient and thorough examination of the lenses of both eyes may yield useful information about the cause of the cataract.

Progressive retinal atrophy is a differential diagnosis to chorioretinitis. In progressive retinal atrophy the changes are always bilateral and symmetrical and there are no signs of inflammatory disease.

Treatment and prognosis

The primary disease must be treated, if the underlying cause of the uveitis can be established. Otherwise, symptomatic treatment (corticosteroids and/or non-steroidal anti-inflammatory drugs and mydriatic–cyclopegic drugs) is indicated. The treatment usually has to be continued for a long period of time, usually months. In some cases it is advisable to maintain topical anti-inflammatory treatment lifelong to avoid recurrence of the uveitis and limit the risk of additional complications. Immunosupressive drugs, for example, azathioprine, have mainly been used in cases unresponsive to conventional therapy, such as uveodermatologic syndrome in dogs [46].

The prognosis depends on the cause and degree of damage to the tissues. Long-term therapeutic success should not be expected in most cases. The prognosis is generally grave in cases with glaucoma secondary to uveitis.

Chronic glaucoma

The condition arises when the earlier signs of glaucoma are neglected or unnoticed or when therapeutic efforts have been insufficient. The damage to the eye is usually considerable. Signs of pain are usually not obvious and chronic glaucomatous eyes often seem to be well tolerated by the patient, although attitude and behaviour frequently improve following therapy.

Clinical signs

Chronic glaucomas share several clinical signs, although various initial causes of the glaucoma are possible. The clinical signs are often less prominent in cats compared to dogs. Pain is usually not conspicuous in chronic stages of glaucoma and the eye is held open. However, concurrent uveitis may cause discomfort.

The most obvious sign is usually enlargement of the globe, buphthalmia. The enlargement takes a long time (months) in adults, but may develop in less than a week in puppies and kittens. It is sometimes difficult to appreciate slight enlargement of the globe in cats. Episcleral blood vessels may or may not look congested, and IOP may vary from normal to elevated. Distended episcleral vessels and normal IOP are most commonly seen in dogs, where the IOP has been considerably elevated for a long time. Corneal changes, for example chronic corneal edema and white irregular streaks, or Haab's striae, are common. Buphthalmia with or without lagophthalmus can cause keratitis and corneal ulcers. The cornea may also be enlarged (megalocornea) in patients with buphthalmia. Gonioscopy usually shows a collapsed ciliary cleft or closed iridocorneal angle with different degrees of peripheral anterior synechia. Development of secondary cataracts and subluxation or luxation of the lens may be present. The possibility of an anteriorly luxated lens should be borne in mind in patients with dense corneal edema. Visible changes in the posterior part of the eye include liquefaction of the vitreous body, various degrees of retinal degeneration, and cupping and atrophy of the optic nerve head. Atrophy and cupping of the optic nerve head is not an obvious feature in cats, because of their normal lack of myelin in the optic nerve. The IOP may be within the normal range in advanced cases.

Diagnosis

Chronic glaucoma is easily diagnosed because the clinical signs are obvious and easily recognized. The initial cause of glaucoma is often impossible to tell, because of abundant secondary changes within the eye. The possibility of concurrent chronic uveitis or ocular neoplasia, the two most common causes of secondary glaucoma in cats [47], must be considered.

Treatment and prognosis

The aim of treatment in most chronic cases is to keep the animal comfortable and pain free. Lowering the IOP to less than 30 mm Hg is usually sufficient to avoid pain and enlargement of the globe. If some vision is still present, it is advisable to try to keep the IOP very low, probably less than 15 mm Hg, to maintain vision and surgical options may be considered. If primary glaucoma is suspected to be the cause of unilateral chronic glaucoma, the unaffected eye may be treated prophylactically [35]. Furthermore, the owner should be advised to monitor the remaining normotensive eye thoroughly and immediately report signs of (acute) glaucoma.

Exposure keratitis, corneal ulcerations, and mechanical injuries as well as concurrent, often low-grade uveitis must be treated symptomatically. Buphthalmic eyes rarely respond well to medical treatment. Procedures reducing aqueous humor production, cyclocryotherapy, laser ablation of the ciliary body, or intravitreal injection of gentamicin may be necessary. Radical surgical procedures, for example enucleation or evisceration, should be considered in eyes with marked buphthalmia. Chemical ablation with gentamicin and the use of evisceration and intraocular prosthesis should not be used in cats, because of the risk of development of ocular sarcoma [48].

Chronic glaucomatous eyes are usually blind. Buphthalmia is an unfavourable sign where the prognosis for vision is concerned, except in young animals, where the condition develops rapidly. Perception of light is sometimes present in patients with advanced chronic changes and some breeds, such as the Norwegian Elkhound, seem to be more resistant to glaucomatous damage than others.

Cataract

The lens is a clear structure of epithelial origin, constantly growing throughout life, as new fibers are formed by elongation of equatorial epithelial cells. The older cells form the nucleus, while the cortex consists of younger cells. The lens fibers meet at the poles, in dogs forming an upright Y anteriorly and an inverted Y posteriorly. The lens is avascular, which precludes typical inflammatory reactions. In general, pathological changes in the lens include hydropic swelling of lens fibers, lysis of fibers and attempted fiber regeneration resulting in epithelial hyperplasia and capsular thickening.

The term cataract is derived from the Greek word *kataruraktes* (waterfall). As a medical term, cataract defines every non-physiologic opacification of lens fibers and/or the capsule, regardless of the etiology.

Cataracts are most easily diagnosed by retroillumination. The lens opacity will present as a dark and more or less opaque area against the brighter fundus reflex. More thorough examination of the lens demands the use of a slit-lamp biomicroscope.

Cataracts can be classified according to stage of development, type, localization, and etiology. In practice, the stage and type are the most important types of classification. The stages of development are incipient, immature, mature, and hypermature.

- *Incipient cataract* describes focal opacification(s) of the lens and/ or its capsule. Vision is not impaired. This cataract may or may not progress.
- *Immature cataract*. The opacity is more or less diffuse, but the fundus can still be examined. Vision may or may not be impaired. The changes are mostly progressive.
- *Mature cataract*. The fundus cannot be inspected, as the opacification is complete and dense. Vision is severely impaired. If a mature cataract takes up fluid and swells it is referred to as intumescent.
- *Hypermature cataract*. Dissolving of the cataract may occasionally occur. The content of the lens capsule is more or less liquefied. Lens protein can be resorbed, leading to shrinkage of the lens with wrinkling and dimpling of the capsule. The nucleus will dissolve to a lesser extent and may migrate inferiorly in the capsular bag to form what is termed a Morgagnian cataract.

If a cataract is present at birth it is considered congenital. Cataracts developing after the eighth week are termed developmental [49]. Senile cataracts may occur in aged animals, but should not be confused with nuclear sclerosis which is a normal ageing process of the lens.

Cataracts are caused by several factors, some of which are:

- Congenital anomalies
- Genetic factors
- Toxins
- Radiation
- Trauma

- Other ocular diseases
- Systemic diseases
- Ageing

Cataracts are also described according to localization within the lens. In animals cataracts are classified as nuclear, anterior or posterior cortical or subcapsular, equatorial, or capsular. Nuclear cataracts most frequently occur in the congenital form. Pulverulent cataract, where the nucleus has a 'candy floss' appearance, is occasionally seen. The condition most often does not progress to disturb vision.

Hereditary cataract

Primary hereditary cataracts have been described in many breeds of dogs and the list is continuously growing. According to the gene pool in different countries, the incidence of hereditary cataracts within a breed may differ significantly. Hereditary cataracts are far more rare in cats, but are suspected in the Persian, Birman, and Himalayan [50].

It may be difficult to determine whether a cataract should be considered hereditary or not. However, the more of the following criteria that are met in conjunction with an affected animal, the greater is the likelihood that the cataract is hereditary:

- Hereditary cataract has previously been described in the breed.
- The cataract occurs bilaterally.
- The age of appearance and the localization of the lenticular changes correspond to those described for the breed.
- The cataract is progressive, although slowly in certain cases.

The problem arises when suspected hereditary forms of cataract are diagnosed in a 'new' breed. Examination of the parents, littermates, and offspring should be performed. Hereditary cataracts may be congenital or developmental.

Congenital hereditary cataract

In congenital hereditary cataract the nucleus and perinuclear cortex are most often affected by the opacification. Congenital cataracts confined to the nucleus are generally non-progressive: cortical involvement is a poor prognosticator. It may occur in combination with other congenital eye abnormalities, such as microphthalmia, retinal dysplasia, PPM, posterior lenticonus/lentiglobus and PHTVL/PHPV. Primary congenital cataracts not associated with malformations of the eye may be seen in breeds like the Staffordshire Bull Terrier, the West Highland White Terrier, and the Boston Terrier.

Congenital cataract associated with microphthalmia is diagnosed

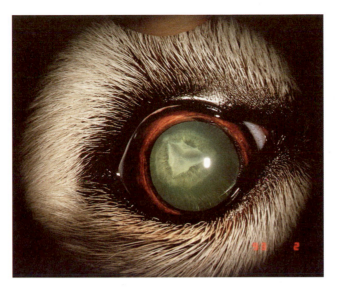

Figure 5.21 Posterior polar cataracts (bilateral) in a 2 year old dog with minor visual problems, according to the owner.

among others in the Miniature Schnauzer, English Cocker Spaniel, Cavalier King Charles Spaniel, West Highland White Terrier and Old English Sheepdog. In the Cavalier King Charles Spaniel, congenital cataract often occurs in combination with lenticonus or lentiglobus. Apart from the cataract in the Miniature Schnauzer, which is inherited autosomal recessively, the mode of inheritance has not been established. It is important to note that not all congenital bilateral cataracts are inherited.

The triangular posterior polar cataract seen in the Golden and Labrador Retrievers as well as other breeds including Rottweilers and Belgian Sheepdogs is considered developmental as it occurs after 6 months of age in most cases (Figure 5.21).

Inherited developmental cataract

Most developmental cataracts begin in the cortex and may progress to involve the whole lens, including the nucleus. The rate of progression varies, from barely noticeable to rapidly progressing changes. The list of breeds with proven or suspected inherited developmental cataract is long, with local variations. Further information on hereditary or suspected hereditary cataracts is available in the literature [19, 20, 51].

Lens-induced uveitis

This problem may accompany both cataract formation and resorbtion. Increased cell content of the aqueous humor has been found in cataracts, indicating a mild inflammation, but without leading to clinically obvious uveitis [52]. However, especially in rapidly progressing and in hypermature cataracts, clinically significant uveitis may be present. This is most often a chronic condition with scleral injection and moderate discomfort. The iris is not extremely swollen, but the chronic condition will eventually result in a darkening of the iris color with or without pupillary cysts. The pupil is slightly constricted, resistant to mydriasis, and the intraocular pressure is lowered. A granulomatosis variant seen most commonly in association with diabetic cataracts is characterized by prominent keratic precipitates and may be refractory to therapy.

Traumatic cataract

Traumatic cataract can develop as a result of blunt trauma or a perforating wound, for instance by a cat claw. Small perforations of the capsule may seal with fibrin and posterior synechiae, with a resultant non-progressive cataract. Blunt trauma or perforating larger wounds may cause more extensive changes, progressing to complete cataracts. Release of lens proteins into the anterior chamber usually results in intense uveitis.

Toxic cataract

Several toxic substances can cause cataracts [53]. These include mitotic agents, enzyme inhibitors, and certain metals. Cataract formation after long-term therapy with ketaconazole has also been described. A brand of commercial milk replacement produced cataracts in orphaned puppies [54], although this type of cataract might be better classified as a nutritional type.

Cataract secondary to other ocular diseases

In a number of other eye diseases, cataract can develop secondarily. Progressive retinal atrophy (PRA) in dogs (not in cats), often results in secondary cataract, obscuring the primary disease. Questioning of the owner about onset, vision in daylight and under reduced lighting conditions, as well as the age and the breed of the dog is of essence to establish a diagnosis. ERG should always be performed before cataract surgery if primary retinal disease is suspected and the retina cannot be visualized ophthalmoscopically.

Uveitis, especially in the cat, frequently leads to cataract formation as do lens luxation and glaucoma. These cataracts are caused by an altered composition of the aqueous humor, which is responsible for lens nutrition.

Cataract secondary to systemic diseases

Diabetes mellitus is a common cause of cataracts and most diabetic dogs eventually develop lens changes [55]. The cataracts are bilateral, rapidly progressive and involve the entire lens. Typical findings in diabetic cataracts are broad and clearly marked suture line separation ('water-cleft' formation). The cause of cataract has been considered to be an increase in glucose in the aqueous. The excess glucose is metabolized via the aldose reductase pathway, resulting in increased concentration of sorbitol. Sorbitol acts as an osmotic agent drawing water into the lens cells, thus causing swelling of the fibers and loss of transparency.

Treatment

Despite anecdotal reports, no effective medical treatment for cataract exists. Atropine eyedrops for pupil dilatation can be worthwhile if the cataract is small and situated in the central visual axis.

Surgical treatment with lens extraction provides predictable restoration of functional vision. The general condition of the patient as to health and behaviour should be considered. Cataract surgery

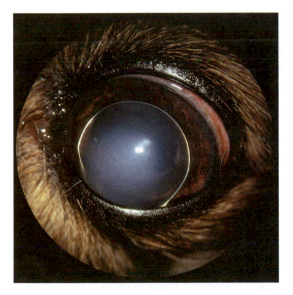

Figure 5.22   Primary anterior lens luxation in a 2 year old Yorkshire Terrier. The lens can be seen in the anterior chamber.

should be left to veterinarians with special interest in ophthalmology and experience in lens extractions.

There are two basic techniques for removal of a cataractous lens: intracapsular or extracapsular lens extraction. In intracapsular extraction the lens is removed *in toto*. That is, the zonular fibers are broken and the lens is removed from the vitreous. There is a high risk of complications, and the method is never used in cats and dogs, except in cases of lens luxation (Figure 5.22). In extracapsular extraction an opening is made in the anterior capsule and the lens contents are removed. The nucleus of the lens is taken out via the corneal incision, with subsequent cleaning of the capsular bag by irrigation and aspiration of residual cortical material. In phacoemulsification, the lens material is fragmented by ultrasound and aspirated. The equipment for phacoemulsification is expensive, but the method offers essential advantages; the trauma to the interior of the eye is less and the corneal incision is not larger than the phaco needle. Both methods of extracapsular lens extraction, however, require careful evaluation before surgery, as well as close follow-up after surgery. Postoperative medication is indicated for several months.

An aphakic (without a lens) animal is strongly hyperopic (far sighted) and the use of intraocular lenses in cataract surgery has gained increased popularity.

The success rate of extracapsular lens extractions varies, depending on the type of cataract, the skill of the surgeon, the method used, and the cooperation of the patient; in general in experienced hands 90% success rates should be anticipated. Frequent usually insignificant complications after cataract surgery are adhesions and capsular fibrosis. Glaucoma, retinal detachment, corneal edema, and endophthalmitis are critical complications that occur less commonly.

Inherited retinal degeneration

Generalized progressive retinal degeneration (PRA)

Classical PRA has been described in a great number of dog breeds as well as in a few cat breeds [19, 20]. The condition has been further clarified through clinical, biochemical, morphological, and electrophysiological studies in several breeds [32] and molecular genetic studies are also in progress in some affected breeds. It is now clear that classical PRA groups together several diseases at the cellular level although the clinical manifestations are more or less similar. Thus, the age of onset of PRA may vary between breeds as well as the progressivity of the retinal disease process. PRA has, furthermore, been grossly divided into two main disease types; PRA of early onset and usually fast progression (such as rod–cone-, rod-, or cone-dysplasia) and late onset PRA, usually with a slow progression of retinal degeneration. In the latter type of PRA the photoreceptors show normal development, but degenerate after the time of retinal maturation, which occurs at about 8 weeks in the dog [56]. A common finding in all types of PRA is that the disease process is always bilateral and always leads to blindness. Through genetic studies an autosomal recessive inheritance for the defect has been demonstrated in all breeds studied except one; the exception is the Siberian Husky where an X-linked disorder has been shown [57]. See Table 5.3 for a summary of specific inherited retinal diseases in dog and cat breeds.

Progressive rod–cone degeneration

In the Miniature Poodle, classical generalized PRA has been further specified as progressive rod–cone degeneration [58, 59]. Morphologically, signs of disease are observed in the Poodle by electron microscopy at the age of 14.5 weeks and at the age of 30 weeks by light microscopy. A reduced renewal rate of outer segment lamellae has been reported as well as abnormal relative concentrations of phospholipids and free fatty acids in rod outer segments. In recent years the retinal degenerative disease in the Toy and Miniature Poodle, English and American Cocker Spaniel, and the Labrador Retriever has been shown to be caused by a mutation at the same gene locus, although the clinical manifestations vary.

The Abyssinian cat is also affected by an autosomal recessively inherited progressive rod–cone degenerative disease [60] with similarities to the Miniature Poodle model described above. Further studies of this specific disease have shown a significant reduction in interphotoreceptor retinol binding protein (IRBP) in affected individuals compared to normals, before signs of retinal degeneration are observed by morphology [61]. It is not clear yet if this is a primary or secondary defect in the photoreceptor disease process.

Clinical findings

Regardless of the specific underlying cause and the age of onset of progressive rod–cone degeneration/generalized PRA, the clinical manifestations tend to be rather similar in affected animals of different breeds. Clinical signs include an initial reduction of night vision, with a successively reduced day and night vision. The end stage is always complete blindness. Early ophthalmoscopic signs are seen as a discoloration of the tapetal fundus (brown to grayish changes most obvious peripherally) with an altered tapetal reflectivity and a slight vascular attenuation between the age of 3–5 years in the Poodle, somewhat earlier in the American Cocker Spaniel, and somewhat later in the English Cocker Spaniel. In the Labrador Retriever there is a great variation in timing of appearance of early retinal changes, between

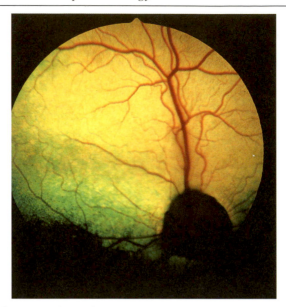

Figure 5.23 Early signs of hereditary rod–cone degeneration (generalized progressive retinal atrophy, PRA) in a 4 year old Labrador Retriever. The dog had slight visual problems at night, but normal day light vision still. Funduscopic changes were minimal, but ERG non-recordable.

the age of 2 years up to 6 years (Figure 5.23). Progression of disease is variable, but a bilateral retinal atrophy is usually observed after another 2–4 years in the affected breeds. ERG is diagnostic between the age of 6–9 months in the Poodle and not until 1.5 years or later in the English Cocker Spaniel and Labrador Retriever breeds. Electro-physiologic findings include low amplitude rod and cone responses, rod responses being more reduced than cone responses initially.

In the affected Abyssinian cat early clinical signs include changes in tapetal reflectivity and grayish lesions centrally near the optic disc and in the peripheral tapetal fundus usually observed between the age of 1.5 to 2 years. The fundal lesions progress to a generalized atrophic fundus with severely attenuated retinal vessels at the age of 3–5 years (Figure 5.24). ERG is diagnostic of the disease after the age of 8 months with significantly reduced rod responses while cone responses are still more or less normal.

Secondary cataracts are usually found in dog breeds affected with progressive rod–cone degeneration/generalized PRA, but not in the cat.

Differential diagnosis

Generalized retinopathy of inflammatory origin is an important differential diagnosis. In most inflammatory retinopathies, however, the

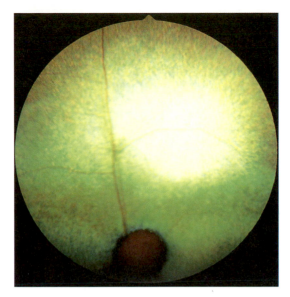

Figure 5.24 Advanced stage of hereditary rod–cone degeneration (PRA) in a 4 year old Abyssinian cat.

retinal changes are not bilaterally symmetrical as in progressive rod–cone degeneration. Furthermore, ERG is often still recordable but is reduced or of small amplitude. Drug-induced retinopathy is, however, difficult to differentiate since retinal changes are often bilateral and symmetrical and there is often a non-recordable ERG. Another differential is SARD. In this disease the onset of clinical signs is acute, with a normal appearing fundus and a non-recordable ERG. But after several months or years of SARD it will be impossible to differentiate this disease clinically from progressive rod–cone degeneration/generalized PRA.

Treatment

There is to date no effective treatment for progressive rod–cone degeneration/generalized PRA in the dog and cat. Preventive measures need to be taken in the breeding programs. Affected animals should not be used for breeding nor should known carriers of the defect, i.e. parents of the affected individual and its offspring in recessive disorders.

Retinal pigment epithelial cell dystrophy (RPED)

In this disease the primary defect is in the pigment epithelial cell layer of the retina. The essential morphologic lesion is hypertrophy of the RPE with accumulation of lipopigments. The defect causes secondary photoreceptor degeneration and retinal atrophy. Because of the clinical appearance of the disease with pigment accumulation and retinal degenerative changes most prevalent in the central part of the retina, this disease was formerly called central progressive retinal atrophy (CPRA) [62]. The disease has been described in several dog breeds particularly the Briard [63], Labrador Retriever, and the Collie breeds. The disease is still widely recognized as having a hereditary basis although there are recent indications that other factors including environmental, may play a significant role in the development and/or expression of the disease.

Clinical findings

Affected dogs usually lose central vision before peripheral vision, with the result that moving objects may still be seen while stationary objects are not. Ophthalmoscopic retinal alterations may be seen from as early as 18 months of age but in some dogs they are not present until much later in life. They appear as light brown pigment foci within the tapetal fundus, usually first developing temporal to the optic disc. With progression of disease the foci become more numerous and may coalesce and areas of hyper-reflectivity develop between them. With advancing disease there is vascular attenuation and more severe retinal atrophic changes and some changes may develop in the non-tapetal fundus such as depigmentation and mottling. The presence or absence of non-tapetal changes appears to vary between affected breeds. Secondary cataract is a common but not consistent finding in older dogs. Usually the changes are bilaterally more or less symmetrical. Affected dogs become severely visually impaired and some become blind. ERG is not diagnostic in RPED. At moderately advanced and advanced stages low-amplitude, barely recordable or non-recordable ERGs are found.

Differential diagnosis

Chorioretinitis can give similar funduscopic changes, although usually not as bilaterally symmetrical as in RPED. In neuronal ceroid lipofuscinosis the fundus appearance may be similar to RPED although, in the former disease, neurological symptoms are usually found as well. Vitamin E deficiency will produce ophthalmoscopic lesions similar to RPED.

Treatment

There is no available treatment to date for RPED. Further studies are needed to elucidate which environmental factors might play a role in the disease process. Also the hereditary basis for the disease needs to

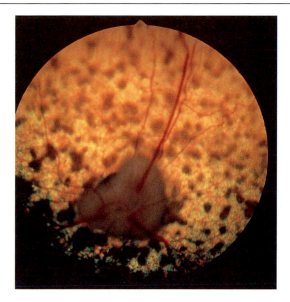

Figure 5.25 Retinal pigment epithelial dystrophy-like lesions in the fundus of a 4 year old Polish Owczarek Nizinni with neuronal ceroid lipofuscinosis.

be clarified. Until this has been done affected individuals should not be used for breeding purposes.

Neuronal ceroid lipofuscinosis

Neuronal ceroid lipofuscinosis has been described in several species [64], including breeds of dogs including the English Setter, Collie, Tibetan Terrier, Dalmation, and Polish Owczarek Nizinni (PON) [65]. The disease is an inborn error of metabolism and causes an accumulation of lipopigments in the brain and in some breeds also in the retina. The retinal lesions are associated with increasing accumulation of autofluorescent and PAS-positive particles of lipopigment in RPE, photoreceptors, and in cells of the inner nuclear layer and the ganglion cells. In the English Setter an autosomal recessive mode of inheritance for the defect has been postulated.

Clinical findings

Blindness, ataxia, and mental disturbances develop at an early age, usually around the age of one year or earlier. The appearance and development of ophthalmoscopic changes varies between breeds. In the PON, funduscopic alterations are obvious at the age of 1–2 years (Figure 5.25), while in the English Setter ophthalmoscopically detectable lesions are absent. ERG is non-recordable (PON) or grossly abnormal with a negative ERG (Tibetan Terrier). The disease leads to death within a few years in the English Setter.

Differential diagnosis

RPED is the main differential with ophthalmoscopic lesions rather similar to the ones observed in neuronal ceroid lipofuscinosis of some breeds, such as in the PON. In RPED the ERG is usually less abnormal than in cases of neuronal ceroid lipofuscinosis. Vitamin E deficiency will also produce ophthalmoscopic lesions similar to RPED and neuronal ceroid lipofuscinosis of the PON breed.

Treatment and prognosis

There is no treatment for affected individuals and the prognosis is poor. Preventive measures should be taken in the breeding of affected individuals and known carriers of the defect.

Nutritional retinal degeneration

Vitamin E deficiency

Vitamin E is an antioxidant with a stabilizing function of cell membranes by the prevention of lipid peroxidation. Deficiency of this vital vitamin in animals may result in pathologic changes in the retina, central nervous system, reproductive tract, and skeletal muscle. Dogs experimentally fed a diet deficient in vitamin E from weaning developed night blindness, ophthalmoscopic fundus changes, and non-recordable ERGs within 4 months [66]. Histologically there was an accumulation of autofluorescent pigment within the RPE and, at later stages, in all retinal layers. Secondary photoreceptor damage was observed with successive development of retinal atrophy. There are obvious similarities between RPED and vitamin E deficiency, which suggest a common etiologic factor.

Vitamin A deficiency

Vitamin A is important for normal visual function. A deficiency is characterized by night blindness in most animals since vitamin A is a precursor of the visual pigment rhodopsin. Vitamin A deficiency is seldom diagnosed in the clinical situation. A deficiency may, however, occur in conjunction with systemic disease resulting in impaired fat absorption. Early changes are characterized by an alteration in color of the tapetal fundus. In a more chronic deficiency there is complete retinal atrophy.

Taurine deficiency retinopathy

Taurine deficiency will cause retinal degeneration (and cardiomyopathy) in the cat [67]. Research has established that taurine, which is a sulphur-containing amino acid, is essential for the cat which has a daily requirement of 35–56 mg [68]. Taurine content is high in milk, liver, and shell-fish, but has been found only at low levels in various dog foods. It is not yet clear if all cases of feline central retinal degeneration (FCRD), the classical name of the disease, are caused by a primary taurine deficiency. It could be that other factors are also involved, such as individual sensitivity to taurine deficiency or problems with absorption of taurine or other required nutrients.

Clinical findings

Ophthalmoscopic evidence for the disease develops after the cat has been on a deficient diet for several months. The signs include bilaterally symmetrical dark grayish lesions in the area centralis. The discolored region enlarges and the center becomes hyper-reflective. With progression the lesion becomes streak-like and is observed along the areas with a high cone density, on both sides of the optic disc (Figure 5.26). Further progression includes a generalized retinopathy with changed reflectivity and vascular attenuation, and the end-stage is complete retinal atrophy. ERG shows reduced amplitudes and

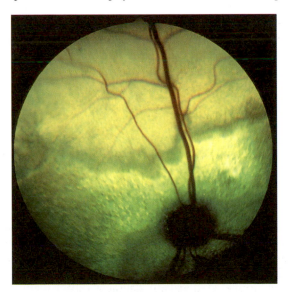

Figure 5.26   A 3 year old European short-haired domestic male cat with moderate to advanced stage of feline central retinal degeneration (FCRD).

increased implicit time of the cone-derived responses early in the disease. With progression of the disorder, ERG is non-recordable.

Differential diagnosis

Generalized retinal atrophy of other causes, such as inflammatory or hereditary, is the main differential to advanced cases of FCRD. The disease cannot be differentiated at this stage since in both cases the animal is blind, pupillary light reflexes are sluggish or absent, and the ERG is non-recordable. Earlier cases of FCRD can be differentiated from chorioretinitis or related disease. In chorioretinitis the lesions are often arbitrarily spread in the fundus and not so typically located as in FCRD.

Treatment and prognosis

Treatment of the disease includes correcting the taurine deficient diet. If this is done before there is a generalized retinopathy there will be no progression of the disorder. In cats already affected with generalized retinal atrophy as a result of taurine deficiency there is no reversibility of the disease.

Posterior segment inflammatory disease

The retina has a high metabolic rate and is nourished from the choriocapillaris and the retinal vasculature. Many disease processes may result in decreased circulation and tissue hypoxia. After hypoxia begins, death of retinal cells follows, intra- and extracellular edema occurs, and neural elements disintegrate with resultant atrophy and gliosis of the retina.

The retina has limited regenerative capacity. Changes in the photoreceptor or other neural elements are often irreversible, limiting the possibilities of treatment of many disorders to prevention of further damage. Lesions of photoreceptors result in secondary loss of inner retinal structures as well as of the retinal vasculature. Trans-synaptic degeneration is less marked in the opposite direction. Chronic lesions of the optic nerve, however, cause degeneration and atrophy of the nerve fiber and ganglion cell layers.

Inflammatory and infectious processes in tissues and structures surrounding the retina, such as vitreous and choroid, may result in severe retinal damage. Examples are autoimmune disorders, bacterial and viral infections as well as neoplastic disorders of the choroid.

The retinal structures react to disease processes as other neural tissues do. In conjunction with inflammation there is an accumulation of cellular debris and edema primarily, thereafter disintegration and degenerative changes prevail, followed by atrophic changes. Ophthalmoscopically these changes appear different depending on fundal

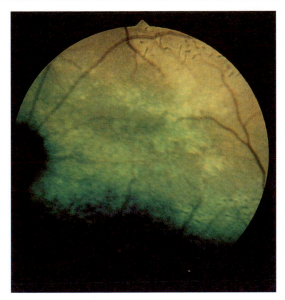

Figure 5.27 Active stage of toxic retinopathy in a young laboratory cat. Inflammatory lesions in the tapetal fundus are grayish. The folding of the neural retina in the peripheral areas is indicative that the inflammation has subsided and that the lesions may be under organization.

area, retinal structures affected, and stage of the inflammatory process. Acute inflammatory lesions in the tapetal fundus appear indistinct, grayish, or dark brown if the neural retina is primarily affected (Figure 5.27). More chronic alterations at this level give a more distinct dark gray or brown color change with or without hyper-reflective regions (Figure 5.28). Long-standing alterations with atrophy of neural retinal structures result in a hyper-reflective tapetal fundus. Acute inflammatory changes in the non-tapetal fundus appear as indistinct, grayish or whitish lesions if the neural retina is affected. In chronic changes there is mainly depigmentation and mottling of the non-tapetal fundus. Inflammatory changes affecting the retinal pigment epithelium look somewhat different in that there is always black or dark brown to gray spots in conjunction with the above described alterations. More chronic alterations affecting the retinal pigment epithelium in the tapetal fundus result in well demarcated pigmented lesions, often in combination with grayish and/or hyperreflective rings around the lesion (Figure 5.28). If the retinal pigment epithelium of the non-tapetal fundus is affected chronically the lesions show up as depigmented areas.

In conjunction with generalized atrophic changes and lack of neural retinal cell tissue there is always an effect on retinal vascu-

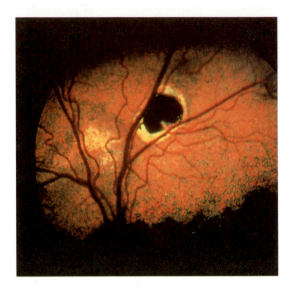

Figure 5.28   Scarring of the tapetal fundus, an incidental finding in a 5 year old Poodle. The lesion to the left is a focal region of inflammation that still may be somewhat active, while the lesion to the right is an inactive lesion with central pigmentation surrounded by hyper-reflectivity, i.e. pigment epithelial hypertrophy with a rim of neural retinal atrophy.

lature, starting with a slight beading of vessels. In generalized disease processes such as in generalized retinopathies of inflammatory or hereditary origin, there is a marked or complete attenuation of retinal vessels.

Chorioretinitis and related conditions

Inflammations affecting the posterior structures of the eye usually involve both choroid and retina concurrently, the choroidal contribution often being predominant. There are several known causes of chorioretinitis and related conditions including bacterial, fungal and viral agents, trauma, neoplasia and foreign bodies. More specifically for the dog some of the recognized causes are; distemper, toxoplasmosis, leishmaniasis, toxocariasis, brucellosis, protothecosis, and oculomycosis (blastomycosis, histoplasmosis, cryptococcosis, coccidiomycosis, and geotrichosis). For the cat identified causes of chorioretinitis and related conditions are feline infectious peritonitis, feline leukemia virus, feline immunodeficiency virus, tuberculosis, toxoplasmosis, and oculomycosis. Nevertheless, many cases of chorioretinitis are idiopathic.

Some causes of retinochoroiditis and chorioretinitis are of public health significance [69]. Toxoplasmosis, caused by *Toxoplasma gondi*, is recognized as a cause of retinal disease in several species, including humans [70]. In this protozoan disease the oocysts are produced by cats and the organism has an intraintestinal cycle that occurs in mammals and birds. Toxocara retinochoroiditis is caused by an ascarid nematode and is an important intestinal parasite in the dog but is of public health significance on account of the possible migration of larvae in humans.

Diagnosis and clinical findings

A general physical examination and laboratory workup is important in all cases of chorioretinitis and related conditions. Affected animals are usually visual; impaired vision usually only results if the inflammatory processes are bilateral and generalized. Pupillary light reflexes and the result of ERG recordings may be normal in chorioretinitis and related conditions. The ophthalmoscopic appearance of the fundus is indicative of an inflammatory process. It is not unusual, in conjunction with routine ophthalmoscopic screening for hereditary retinal disease, to find chronic focal lesions in the fundus (retinal scars) (Figure 5.28), sequelae to low-grade chorioretinitis, with no clinical significance to the animal.

Differential diagnosis

An important differential to chorioretinitis is RPED. In the latter disease, retinal lesions are generalized and bilateral, which is not always the case with chorioretinitis. Another differential is multifocal RD particularly in the English Springer Spaniel, in which the lesions may be difficult to differentiate from chorioretinitis. In the former disease, however, the lesions, are most often found centrally in the tapetal fundus, often along or in the vicinity of the larger superior vessels. In multifocal RD, the funduscopic lesions are, furthermore, often curvilinear or small and circular while in chorioretinitis the changes are often larger and more darkly pigmented and often with hyper-reflective areas or circles around a darkly pigmented spot. The end stage of generalized retinal atrophy may also be difficult to differentiate from generalized chorioretinitis lesions. Most often the former is bilaterally symmetrical, while the latter rarely is. Histopathology may help to provide the correct diagnosis in such cases.

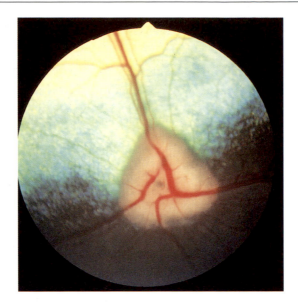

Figure 5.29   Papilledema in a 2 year old acutely blind Norwegian Elkhound. The dog had no other clinical signs. Autopsy revealed a tumor in the optic chiasm.

Treatment

The primary cause should be treated. The use of systemic antimicrobials is useful in most ·cases while corticosteroids may be contraindicated in cases of active infections. Diuretics may be of value in cases of severe retinal edema or detachments.

Optic nerve disease

The optic nerve consists of the myelinated axons of the retinal ganglion cells before they exit from the globe through the cribriform plate of the sclera. The optic nerve may be affected by developmental abnormalities, either inherited or non-inherited, trauma, neoplasia, and inflammatory processes in the nerve or its adnexa. Primary chronic lesions of the optic nerve, which often result in atrophic changes in the nerve, also cause retrograde changes such as degeneration and atrophy of the nerve fiber and ganglion cell layers of the retina.

Papilledema

Papilledema is a non-inflammatory swelling of the optic disc and is usually caused by increased pressure on the optic nerve. This occurs in conjunction with brain tumors in the region of the optic chiasm (Figure 5.29) [71] and sometimes also in systemic hypertension.

Papilledema itself does not impair vision and pupillary light reflexes are present, and the ERG is normal. Ophthalmoscopically the optic disc appears enlarged but there are no inflammatory components. If the papilledema is not controlled through treatment of the primary disease, the optic nerve head will atrophy, which results in blindness.

Chronic neurologic disorders causing blindness

This group of diseases rarely shows visual impairment as the only clinical sign, although apparent blindness may be the only indication of disease noted by the owner. A general and neurologic examination usually reveals other signs of abnormal function. Localization of the site of the deficit in the visual pathway should be attempted.

For a thorough description of neurologic diseases causing blindness, the reader is recommended to read textbooks on neurology. However, the most important diseases will be briefly mentioned here.

Hepatic encephalopathy

Hepatic encephalopathy is an endogenous intoxication, a complex metabolic disorder resulting from liver dysfunction. The condition may develop either because of advanced liver damage, or secondary to portosystemic venous shunts, which divert portal blood past the liver into the caudal vein [72]. Potentially toxic products absorbed in the gastrointestinal tract are normally detoxified in the liver, but in the present condition they enter the systemic circulation instead. These toxic products include ammonia which is produced by bacteria in the colon and normally converted to urea in the liver, as well as dietary amino acids usually metabolized in the liver. Ammonia and certain amino acids may act as neurotoxins to the brain.

Clinical findings and diagnosis

Clinical signs are most confusing in young animals with congenital portosystemic shunts. The animals may present apparently blind, especially shortly after a meal consisting of food with high protein levels. Other signs, such as excitation or confusion, may also be present. Diagnosis is established by blood chemistry, urinalysis, and imaging techniques for liver tissue and vessels.

Treatment and prognosis

In chronic liver damage, supportive treatment, including a low-protein diet, is recommended. If the condition is caused by vascular abnormalities, identification and closing of the shunting vein(s) before secondary liver disease develops is the recommended treatment.

Lysosomal storage disease

These rare conditions are often genetic and may affect both dogs and cats [73]. Lysosomal storage diseases include diseases in which the absence of a specific enzyme leads to the accumulation of its substrates with subsequent cell damage, or the disease may be a direct result of the metabolic disturbance. Many enzymes in cells are contained within small organelles called lysosomes. The enzymes are involved in a variety of catabolic processes and in tissue or substrate turnover (mainly degradation) pathways in the CNS. Because the retina and retinal pigment epithelium are of neuroectodermal origin, they can also be involved in these diseases. Fundus changes, due to accumulation of degraded material, followed by degeneration, may be diagnosed. Lysosomal enzyme deficiencies fall into several groups; glycogen storage diseases, glycolipid catabolism diseases, ceroid–lipofuscin storage diseases, and mucopolysaccharidoses.

Clinical findings

Onset of clinical signs is usually in the first months of life. The diseases are slowly progressive in nature, most often leading to the death of the animal. The degenerative changes are diffuse and, like in other CNS diseases, blindness may be the initial complaint. In cats, other findings, including facial abnormalities and corneal cloudiness, may accompany the CNS signs.

Treatment

No treatment exists in these diseases. As most of the diseases are recessively inherited, affected animals, their offspring, and parents should not be used for breeding.

Neoplasms

Primary tumors of the globe are most often melanomas or melanosarcomas arising from the uvea, but tumors originating from other tissues within the eye are also reported [74]. Melanotic tumors are locally expansive with low metastatic potential in the dog, while in cats they may be highly malignant.

While malignant lymphoma is the most common metastatic neoplasm that involves the eye, any malignant tumor may spread to the eye.

Visual pathway abnormalities are often helpful for localizing intracranial tumors. Tumors affecting them may be primary or metastatic. Primary tumors usually grow slowly, but the visual loss may appear to be rather acute. This happens because tumors are space occupying and may grow to a certain size before clinical signs develop. Edema of surrounding tissues is also frequent. Neoplasms may arise within the tissue of the visual pathway itself, or may be space occupying tumors from adjacent structures, compressing vital tissue. Metastatic tumors may have a more acute progression than primary tumors and may be multifocal.

Clinical findings

Many animals may have demonstrated vague signs, such as behavioural changes, for some time before showing more obvious neurologic signs. When blindness related to the CNS is suspected, a thorough neurologic examination should be performed, in particular testing all ocular reflexes and reactions. In addition to signs related to the localization of the lesion, signs related to an increase in intracranial pressure are frequently present, resulting in head pressing and altered behaviour. Papilledema may be seen in some animals but is difficult to evaluate, especially in dogs, because of the great variation in myelination of the optic nerve head.

Pituitary tumors may compress the optic nerves, as well as other cranial nerves. Brain stem tumors are characterized by abnormal gait and cranial nerve signs, including the cranial nerves associated with vision, eye reflexes, and eye movements. Behavioural changes and seizures are usually absent in tumors of the brain stem until the mass affects the reticular activating system (the reticular formation dorsal to the brain stem giving impulses to the cerebral cortex) or alters intracranial pressure.

Ocular abnormalities associated with brain tumors may present as nystagmus, central blindness, pupillary light reflex abnormalities, or abnormal eye movements.

Therapy and prognosis

The signs accompanying brain tumors are often temporarily relieved by corticosteroid and/or anticonvulsant therapy, and some animals with slowly growing tumors may be kept relatively free of clinical signs for several months with such therapy. Radiation therapy and surgery, when possible, may provide therapeutic options, but the prognosis is grave.

REFERENCES

1. Farris BK. *The Basics of Neuro-ophthalmology*, St. Louis: Mosby Year Book 1991.

2. Oliver JE and Lorenz MD. *Handbook of Veterinary Neurology*, 2nd edn. Philadelphia: WB Saunders 1993.

3. Murphy CJ, Zadnik K and Mannis MJ. Myopia and refractive error in dogs. *Invest. Ophthalmol. Vis. Sci.* 1992; **33**: 2459–63.

4. Acland GM. Diagnosis and differentiation of retinal diseases in small animals by electroretinography. *Semin. Vet. Med. Surg.* (Small Anim). 1988; **3**: 15–27.

5. Gouras P. Electroretinography: Some basic principles. *Invest. Ophthalmol.* 1970; **9**: 557–69.

6. Granit R. The components of the retinal action potential in mammals and their relation to the discharge in the optic nerve. *J. Physiol.* 1933; **77**: 207–39.

7. Aguirre G. Rod and cone contributions to the canine electroretinogram. *Ph.D. thesis*: University of Pennsylvania, 1975.

8. Narfström K, Andersson B-E, Andreasson S and Gouras P. Clinical electroretinography in the dog using Ganzfeld stimulation: A practical method of examining rod and cone function. *Doc. Ophthalmol.* 1995; **90**: 279–90.

9. Sims MH, Loratta LJ, Bubb WJ and Morgan RV. Waveform analysis and reproducibility of visual-evoked potential in dogs. *Am. J. Vet. Res.* 1989; **50**: 1823–28.

10. Barnett KC and Knight GC. Persistent pupillary membrane and associated defects in the basenji. *Vet. Rec.* 1969; **85**: 242–9.

11. Strande A, Nicolaissen B and Bjerkås I. Persistent pupillary membrane and congenital cataract in a litter of Engish Cocker Spaniels. *J. Small Anim. Pract.* 1988; **29**: 257–60.

12. Stades FC. Persistant hyperplastic tunica vasculosa lentis and persistant hyperplastic primary vitreous (PHTVL/PHPV) in the Dobermann Pinscher. *Ph.D. thesis*: Government University of Utrecht 1983.

13. Narfström K and Dubielzig R. Posterior lenticonus, cataracts and microphthalmia; congenital ocular defects in the Cavalier King Charles Spaniel. *J. Small Anim. Pract.* 1984; **25**: 669–77.

14. Narfström K. Cataract in the West Highland White Terrier. *J. Small Anim. Pract.* 1981; **22**: 467–71.

15. Leon A. Diseases of the vitreous in the dog and cat. *J. Small Anim. Pract.* 1988; **29**: 448–61.

16. Boevé MH and Stades FC. Persistent hyperplastic tunica vasculosa lentis and primary vitreous in the dog. A comparative review. *Prog. Vet. Comp. Ophthalmol.* 1992; **2**: 163–72.

17. Leon A, Curtis R and Barnett KC. Hereditary persistent hyperplastic primary vitreous in the Staffordshire Bull Terrier. *J. Am. Anim. Hosp. Ass.* 1986; **22**: 765–74.

18. Whiteley HE. Dysplastic canine retinal morphogenesis. *Invest Ophthalmol. Vis. Sci.* 1991; **32**: 1492–98.

19. The ACVO Genetics Committee. *Ocular Disorders Proven or Suspected to be Hereditary in Dogs*, American College of Veterinary Ophthalmologists 1992.

20. Rubin LF. *Inherited Eye Diseases in the Purebred Dog*, Baltimore: Williams & Wilkins 1989.

21. Yakely WL, Wyman M, Donovan EF and Fechheimer NS. Genetic

transmission of an ocular fundus anomaly in collies. *J. Am. Vet. Med. Ass.* 1968; **152**: 457–61.

22. Wyman M, Donovan EF. Eye anomaly of the collie. *J. Am. Vet. Med. Ass.* 1969; **165**: 866–70.

23. Barrie KP, Lavach JD and Gelatt KN. Diseases of the canine posterior segment. In: Gelatt KN (ed) *Textbook of Veterinary Ophthalmology*, Philadelphia: Lea & Febiger 1981: 480–83.

24. Bjerkås E. Collie eye anomaly in the rough collie in Norway. *J. Small Anim. Pract.* 1991; **32**: 89–92.

25. Aguirre GD, Farber DB, Lolley R et al. Retinal degenerations in the dog. III. Abnormal cyclic nucleotide metabolism in rod–cone dysplasia. *Exp. Eye Res.* 1982; **35**: 625–42.

26. Suber ML, Pittler SJ, Quin N *et al.* Irish setter dogs affected with rod–cone dysplasia contain a nonsense mutation in the rod cGMP phosphodiesterase beta-subunit gene. *Proc. Natl. Acad. Sci. USA* 1993; **90**: 3968–72.

27. Clements PJM, Gregory CY, Petersen-Jones SM *et al.* Confirmation of the rod cGMP phosphodiesterase beta-subunit (PDEβ) nonsense mutation in affected rcd-1 Irish setters in the UK and development of a diagnostic test. *Curr. Eye Res.* 1993; **12**: 861–6.

28. Ray K, Baldwin VJ, Acland GM *et al.* Cosegregation of codon 807 mutation of the canine rod cGMP phosphodiesterase β gene and rcd1. *Invest. Ophthalmol. Vis. Sci.* 1994; **35**: 4291–9.

29. Petersen-Jones SM, Clements PJM, Barnett KC *et al.* Incidence of the gene mutation causal for rod–cone dysplasia type 1 in Irish setters in the UK. *J. Small Anim. Pract.* 1995; **36**: 310–14.

30. Aguirre GD. Retinal degenerations in the dog: I. Rod dysplasia. *Exp. Eye Res.* 1978; **26**: 233–53.

31. Acland GM and Aguirre GD. Retinal degenerations in the dog. IV. Early retinal degeneration (erd) in Norwegian Elkhounds. *Exp. Eye Res.* 1987; **44**: 491–521.

32. Parshall CJ, Wyman M, Nitroy S, Acland G and Aguirre G. Photoreceptor dysplasia: An inherited progressive retinal dystrophy of miniature Schnauzer dogs. *Prog. Vet. Comp. Ophthalmol.* 1991; **1**: 187–203.

33. Narfström K, Wrigstad A, Ekesten B and Nilsson SEG. Hereditary retinal dystrophy in the Briard dog: clinical and hereditary characteristics. *Prog. Vet. Comp. Ophthalmol.* 1994; **4**: 85–92.

34. Aguirre GD and Rubin LF. The electroretinogram in dogs with inherited cone degeneration. *Invest. Ophthalmol.* 1975; **14**: 840–47.

35. Slater MR and Erb HN. Effects of risk factors and prophylactic treatment on primary glaucoma in the dog. *J. Am. Vet. Med. Ass.* 1986; **188**: 1028–30.

36. Martin C, Kaswan R, Gratzek A, Champagne E, Salisbury M-A and Ward D. Ocular use of tissue plasminogen activator in companion animals. *Prog. Vet. Comp Ophthalmol.* 1993; **3**: 29–36.

37. van der Woerdt A, Nasisse MP and Davidson MG. Sudden acquired retinal degeneration in the dog: clinical and laboratory findings in 36 cases. *Prog. Vet. Comp. Ophthalmol.* 1991; **1**: 11–18.

38. Peiffer Jr. RL, Monticello T and Bouldin TW. Primary ocular sarcomas in the cat. *J. Small Anim. Pract.* 1988; **29**: 105–16.

39. Kaswan RL, Bounous D and Hirsh SG. Diagnoses and medical management of keratoconjunctivitis sicca. *Cyclosporine: Veterinary Application in Ophthalmic Disease*, Veterinary Learning Systems Co. 1994: 21–30.
40. Chavkin MJ, Roberts SM, Salman MD, Severin GA and Scholten NJ. Risk factors for development of chronic superficial keratitis in dogs. *J. Am. Vet. Med. Ass.* 1994; **204**: 1630–4.
41. Clerc B. Chronic superficial keratitis in German Shepherd dogs. *Cyclosporine: Veterinary Application in Ophthalmic Disease*, Veterinary Learning Systems Co. 1994: 48–54.
42. Clerc B and Jegou JP. Superficial punctate keratitis. *Cyclosporine: Veterinary Application in Ophthalmic Disease*, Veterinary Learning Systems Co. 1994: 67–71.
43. Crispin SM. Ocular manifestations of hyperlipoproteinaemia. *J. Small Anim. Pract.* 1993; **34**: 500–6.
44. Crispin SM. The pre-ocular tear film and conditions of the conjunctiva and cornea. In: Petersen-Jones SM & Crispin SM (eds) *Manual of Small Animal Ophthalmology*, London: BSAVA Publications 1993: 137–72.
45. Olin DD. Examination of the aqueous humor as a diagnostic aid in anterior uveitis. *J. Am. Vet. Med. Ass.* 1977; **171**: 557–9.
46. Morgan RV. Vogt-Koyanagi-Harada syndrome in humans and dogs. *Comp. Cont. Educ. Pract. Vet.* 1989; **11**: 1211–1218.
47. Wilcock BP and Peiffer Jr. RL, Davidson MG. The causes of glaucoma in cats. *Vet. Pathol.* 1990; **27**: 35–40.
48. Peiffer Jr. RL. Intraocular gentamicin in glaucoma (Letter). *Vet. Comp. Ophthalmol.* 1994; **4**: 166.
49. Stades FC. Diseases of the lens and vitreous. In: Kirk RW (ed) *Current Veterinary Therapy IX*, Philadelphia: W.B. Saunders 1986: 660–69.
50. Hoskins JD. Congenital defects of cats. *Comp. Cont. Educ. Pract. Vet.*, 1995; **17**: 385–405.
51. Petersen-Jones SM. Conditions of the lens. In: Petersen-Jones SM and Crispin SM (eds) *Manual of Small Animal Ophthalmology*, London: BSAVA Publications 1993: 213–28.
52. Krohne SG and Krohne DT. Use of laser flaremetry to measure aqueous humor protein concentrations in dogs. *J. Am. Vet. Med. Ass.* 1995; **206**: 1167–82.
53. Martin CL, Christmas R and Leipold HW. Formations of temporary cataracts in dogs given a dispophenol preparation. *J. Am. Vet. Med. Ass.* 1972; **161** 294–301.
54. Glaze MB and Blanchard GL. Nutritional cataracts in a Samoyed litter. *J. Am. Anim. Hosp. Ass.* 1983; **19**: 951–3.
55. Bagley LH and Lavach JD. Comparisons of postoperative phacoemulsification results in dogs with and without diabetes mellitus: 153 cases (1991–1992). *J. Am. Vet. Med. Ass.* 1994; **205**: 1165–9.
56. Gum GG, Gelatt KN and Samuelsson DA. Maturation of the canine neonate as determined by electroretinography and histology. *Am. J. Vet. Res.* 1984; **45**: 1166–71.
57. Hershfield B, Micklethwaite C, Mullings SJ, Blanton SH, Acland GM and Aguirre GD. RFLP mapping of x-linked progressive retinal atrophy (XLPRA) in the Siberian Husky. *Invest. Ophthalmol. Vis. Sci.* 1994; **35**: 1612.

58. Aguirre GD, Alligood J, O'Brien P and Buyukmihci N. Pathogenesis of progressive rod–cone degeneration in miniature poodles. *Invest. Ophthalmol. Vis. Sci.* 1982; **23**: 610–30.
59. Aguirre GD and O'Brien P. Morphological and biochemical studies of canine progressive rod–cone degeneration. *Invest. Ophthalmol. Vis. Sci.* 1986; **27**: 635–55.
60. Narfström K. Retinal degeneration in a strain of Abyssinian cats: A hereditary, clinical, electrophysiological and morphological study. *Ph.D. thesis*: Linköping University and Swedish University of Agricultural Sciences 1985.
61. Wiggert B, van Veen T, Kutty G, et al. An early decrease in interphotoreceptor retinoid-binding protein gene expression in Abyssinian cats homozygous for hereditary rod–cone degeneration. *Cell Tissue Res.* 1994; **278**: 291–8.
62. Barnett KC. Canine retinopathies. III. The other breeds. *J. Small Anim. Pract.* 1965; **6**: 185–96.
63. Bedford PGC. Retinal pigment epithelial dystrophy (CPRA): study of the disease in the Briard. *J. Small Anim. Pract.* 1984; **25**: 129–38.
64. Koppang N. English Setter model and juvenile ceroid-lipofuscinosis in man. *Am. J. Med. Genet.* 1992; **42**: 599–604.
65. Wrigstad A, Nilsson SEG, Dubielzig R and Narfström K. Neuronal ceroid lipofuscinosis in the Polish Owczarek Nizinny (PON) dog. A retinal study. *Doc. Ophthalmol.* 1995; **91**: 33–47.
66. Riis R, Sheffy BE, Loewe E, Kern TJ and Smith JS. Vitamin E deficiency retinopathy of dogs. *Am. J. Vet. Res.* 1981; **42**: 74–86.
67. Hayes KC, Rabin AR and Berson EL. An ultrastructural study of nutritionally induced and reversed retinal degeneration in cats. *Am. J. Pathol.* 1975; **78**: 505.
68. Burger IH and Barnett KC. The taurine requirement of the adult cat. *J. Small Anim. Pract.* 1982; **23**: 533–7.
69. Curtis R, Barnett KC and Leon AL. Diseases of the canine posterior segment. In Gelatt KN (ed) Veterinary Ophthalmology, 2nd edn. Philadelphia: Lea & Febiger 1991.
70. Frenkel JK, Dubey JP and Miller NL. Toxoplasma gondii in cats: Fecal stages identified as coccidian oocysts. *Science* 1970; **167** 893.
71. Palmer AC, Malinowski W and Barnett KC. Clinical signs including papilledema associated with brain tumors in twenty-one dogs. *J. Small Anim. Pract.* 1974; **15**: 359–86.
72. Vulgamott J. Portosystemic shunts. *Vet. Clin. North Am. (Small Anim. Pract.)* 1985; **15**: 229–42.
73. Jolly RD, Palmer DN, Studdert VP, et al. Canine Ceroid-lipofuscinoses: A review and classification. *J. Small Anim. Pract.* 1994; **35**: 299–306.
74. Dubielzig RR. Ocular neoplasia in small animals. *Vet. Clin. North Am. (Small Anim. Pract.)* 1990; **20**: 837–48.

6

Orbital and Ocular Pain

Peter W Renwick and Simon M Petersen-Jones

Pain is a common and important feature of many ocular and orbital diseases. The resulting clinical signs depend on the severity of the pain and include blepharospasm, increased lacrimation and, in more severe cases, even depression and inappetence. Some of the differentials to consider when an animal presents with a painful eye are listed below:

Orbital disease

- Orbital cellulitis/retrobulbar abscess
- Orbital trauma
- Eosinophilic myositis

Eyelid abnormalities

- Entropion
- Blepharitis/eyelid abscessation
- Ectopic cilia
- Other cilia abnormalities

Ocular surface disease

- Trauma
- Corneal ulceration

Intraocular disease

- Acute uveitis
- Glaucoma (especially acute)
- Anterior lens luxation

ORBITAL DISEASE AS A CAUSE OF PAIN

The orbit of cats and dogs is only partially enclosed by bone meaning that:

- Opening the mouth is painful in animals with orbital inflammatory disease due to pressure from the vertical ramus of the mandible on orbital contents
- Infection and foreign bodies from the oral cavity may reach the orbit
- The orbit may be accessed for the drainage of retrobulbar abscesses via the mouth (see Figure 6.1).

Careful examination of the animal with painful orbital disease should guide the veterinarian to the correct diagnosis. Rostral dis-

(a)

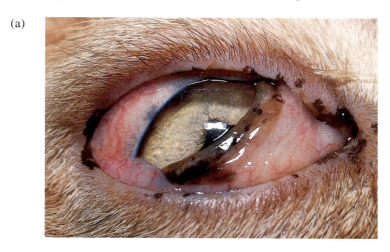

(b)

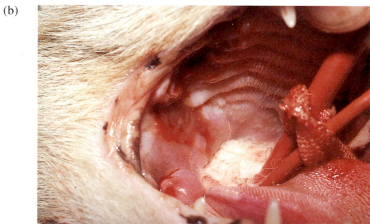

Figure 6.1   (a) A cat with a retrobulbar abscess resulting in exophthalmos, third eyelid protrusion, and conjunctival hyperemia/congestion and swelling. (b) Draining of the retrobulbar abscess in the same cat after blunt dissection to the orbit via the oral mucosa caudal to the last upper molar tooth.

placement of the globe (exophthalmos) is a common feature of several orbital disorders [1, 2]. Exophthalmos is most readily appreciated by viewing the head from above. A comparison of the degree to which the globes can be repelled into the orbit is helpful in deciding if an orbital swelling or space-occupying lesion is present (this will be acutely painful in animals with orbital infection).

Orbital cellulitis/retrobulbar abscess

Orbital infection may result from penetrating wounds (e.g. via the conjunctival sac, eyelids, or mouth), extension from adjacent structures, or possibly hematologic spread. The following signs may result (Figure 6.1):

- Rapid onset of exophthalmos
- Pain, especially on opening mouth (inappetance and depression may result)
- Pyrexia, often accompanied by neutrophilia with a left shift
- Variable facial and adnexal swelling, possibly accompanied by discharging tracts
- Protrusion of the third eyelid
- Conjunctival swelling (chemosis) and hyperemia
- Hyperemia and swelling of the oral mucosa caudal to last molar tooth on the affected side.

Investigation

The clinical features are often diagnostic but a complete blood count (CBC) may be useful. Ultrasonography may enable localization of any pockets of pus. Radiography is usually unrewarding but should be undertaken if a foreign body is suspected or structures adjacent to the orbit are possibly involved. Examination of the oral cavity for areas of inflammation, penetrating wounds, or foreign bodies should be performed and general anesthesia is usually required.

Treatment

Retrobulbar abscesses may be drained via a stab incision through the oral mucosa behind the last molar tooth followed by careful blunt dissection dorsally towards the orbit. Discrete pockets of pus are not always found, but when present samples should be collected for culture and sensitivity (Figure 6.1). A course of broad spectrum systemic antibiotic is provided and reviewed once the bacterial sensitivity results are available. Cellulitis is similarly treated with broad spectrum antibiotics. If there is a lack of response to treatment or recurrence of signs the possibility of the presence of a pocket of pus requiring drainage, or a foreign body necessitating exploratory surgery should be considered.

Eosinophilic myositis

Myositis of the masticatory muscles (eosinophilic myositis) is commonest in young dogs and initially results in painful swelling of the masticatory musculature. Exophthalmos may develop due to swelling of the temporal and pterygoid musculature and is often bilateral. It is accompanied by protrusion of the third eyelid and a reduced range of jaw movement.

Investigation

The signalment and clinical signs in acute cases help in reaching a diagnosis. In chronic cases atrophy of the musculature occurs with resulting enophthalmos. The blood count in some dogs reveals a mild leukocytosis, neutrophilia, and eosinophilia and serum creatinine kinase may be moderately elevated. Histologic examination of muscle biopsies (the temporalis muscle is readily accessed) aid in the diagnosis.

Treatment

The condition is treated with systemic corticosteroids.

Traumatic orbital disease

Injuries affecting the orbit and orbital contents may result from blunt or sharp trauma. There may be associated fractures or penetration of foreign bodies. Proptosis of the globe, which is defined as a forward displacement of the globe beyond the plane of the eyelids, may result from trauma and is considered on p. 56–57.

Investigation

A full clinical examination is mandatory as other injuries may be present. Skull radiographs may be necessary depending on the degree of trauma, or if a radiopaque foreign body is suspected.

Treatment

The treatment required depends on the extent and severity of the lesions.

EYELID ABNORMALITIES AS A CAUSE OF OCULAR PAIN OR IRRITATION

Abnormal eyelid position

Entropion

Entropion [3] is an inward turning of the eyelid leading to contact between the hairy eyelid skin and the ocular surface with resultant irritation or pain and, potentially, corneal damage. It is relatively common in dogs (Figure 6.2) but occurs less frequently in cats (Figure 6.3). It may result from anatomic abnormalities of eyelid and eyelid/globe relationship or it may develop secondarily to blepharospasm resulting from painful ocular surface disorders. The anatomic predispositions are often breed related and the resulting entropion usually affects younger dogs. In the Shar Pei entropion may occur in young puppies and is related to excessive folding of the skin on the head. As the puppies grow the tendency towards entropion decreases. In such cases a temporary eversion of the eyelids using tacking sutures may be all that is necessary (Figure 6.4) [4].

Entropion in juvenile or young adult dogs such as that seen in retrievers, pointers, setters etc. usually requires permanent correction. This is most easily performed by removing a strip of skin or

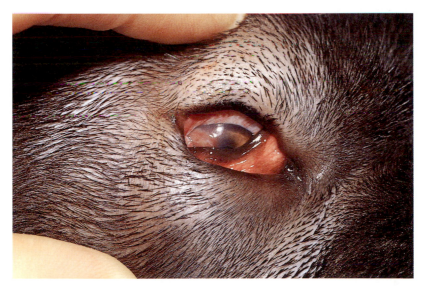

Figure 6.2 Entropion in a Shar Pei. Although the lids are being held open the tendency for the lower eyelid to turn in can be clearly seen. Note the superficial ulceration and vascularization resulting from the abrasion of eyelid hair.

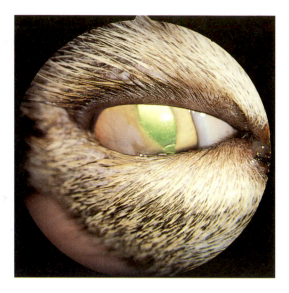

Figure 6.3 Lower eyelid entropion in a cat.

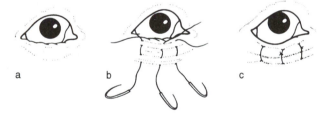

Figure 6.4 Temporary eversion of the lower eyelid to treat entropion in a puppy. (a) The lower eyelid is exhibiting entropion. (b), (c) Two or three temporary everting sutures are placed and tightened sufficiently to correct the entropion. (Redrawn with permission from: Petersen-Jones SM and Crispin SM (eds) *Manual of Small Animal Ophthalmology*, Cheltenham: British Small Animal Veterinary Association Publications 1993).

skin/muscle parallel to and about 3–4mm from the inverted eyelid margin (Figure 6.5). When assessing the degree of correction required, care should be taken to avoid pulling on the skin of the head and thus altering the eyelid position. It is also useful to apply a topical anesthetic to relieve the blepharospastic component, facilitating judgment of the amount of skin to remove to eliminate the actual lid deformity without over correcting.

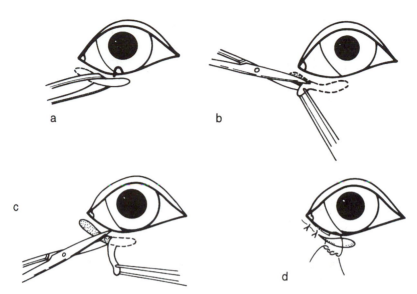

Figure 6.5   Diagram of skin-muscle resection for lower eyelid entropion. (a) The degree of correction has been assessed in the conscious, unsedated animal. Forceps can be used to 'tent up' a ridge of skin corresponding to the amount to be excised. (b) and (c) A strip of skin about 3 mm from the eyelid margin is excised and corresponds to the length of eyelid that is turning in. The width of skin that needs to be removed is governed by the amount that the eyelid turns in. (d) 6/0 sutures are used to repair the skin, the knots should be directed away from the cornea. (Redrawn with permission from: Petersen-Jones SM and Crispin SM (eds) *Manual of Small Animal Ophthalmology*, Cheltenham: British Small Animal Veterinary Association Publications 1993).

Atonic entropion/trichiasis

This condition is most commonly seen in middle aged and older English cocker spaniels. It results from a loss of elasticity of the skin on the head resulting in a slipped facial mask with a rolling in of the upper eyelids so that the eyelashes are in contact with the corneal surface (Figure 6.6). The more severely affected dogs also have a marked lower eyelid ectropion. There is often accompanying chronic pathology including blepharitis, conjunctivitis, keratitis, and corneal ulceration. A reduction in tear production may also develop and contributes to the ocular surface pathology and the general discomfort. Surgical correction is required and the technique described by Stades [5] gives consistently good results (Figure 6.7)

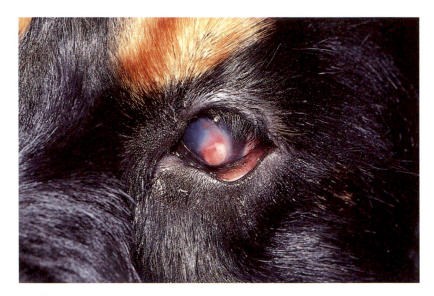

Figure 6.6   Upper eyelid entropion/trichiasis in a middle-aged English Cocker Spaniel. Abrasion from the upper eyelid cilia has caused an area of ulcerative keratitis.

Abnormalities of cilia

Distichiasis

The presence of cilia emerging from the eyelid margin is known as distichiasis. This is a very common finding in dogs, particularly of certain breeds, but is rare in cats. The vast majority of dogs with distichiasis show few signs of irritation. Corneal damage and accompanying pain may occur in a few affected individuals if the cilia are thick and are directed onto the cornea. The management of distichiasis is described on p. 215.

Ectopic cilia

Ectopic cilia are less common than distichia. Similarly to distichia they arise from follicles in or adjacent to the meibomian glands. However, in the case of ectopic cilia they emerge through the conjunctival lining of the eyelid, most commonly singly and typically halfway along the upper eyelid. They almost invariably cause marked discomfort. Usually they occur in young dogs although they may develop in mature dogs, possibly due to metaplasia of the meibomian gland epithelium. Often an area of keratitis or even ulceration develops corresponding to the position of the offending cilium. Magnification is required to see the ectopic cilium and even then it may be hard

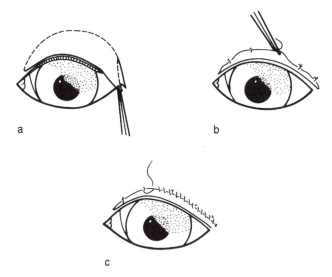

Figure 6.7   Correction of upper eyelid trichiasis/entropion using the technique described by Stades [5]. (a) A skin incision is made 1 mm dorsal to the meibomian gland openings so as to include all the hair bearing skin and extending 3–4 mm lateral to the medial canthus to 5–10 mm past the lateral canthus. The ends of the incision are joined by a second more dorsally positioned incision creating a strip of skin approximately 15–20 mm wide. This strip of skin is removed and any remaining hair follicles excised. (b) The upper skin edge is pulled part way across the wound to approximately the base of the meibomian glands and sutured into place. (c) A continuous suture pattern finishes the repair. The uncovered portion of the wound heals by second intention and creates a narrow strip of hairless skin adjacent to the upper eyelid helping to prevent recurrence of the trichiasis. (Redrawn with permission from: Petersen-Jones SM and Crispin SM (eds) *Manual of Small Animal Ophthalmology*, Cheltenham: British Small Animal Veterinary Association Publications 1993).

to see, particularly if non-pigmented. Treatment consists of removal or destruction of the originating follicle. Destruction may be achieved by cryosurgery or electrolysis; alternatively the follicle may be removed by excising a small block of partial thickness eyelid tissue surrounding the cilium as shown in Figure 6.8.

OCULAR SURFACE LESIONS AS A CAUSE OF PAIN

Corneal ulceration and injury

A corneal ulcer is a lack of continuity in the corneal epithelium, which may or may not be accompanied by stromal loss. The anterior cornea is well supplied with sensory nerve endings and therefore

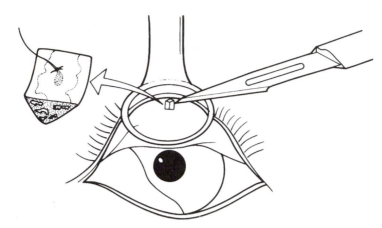

Figure 6.8   Excision of an ectopic cilium. A chalazion clamp immobilizes and everts the upper lid and reduces hemorrhage. A square of partial-thickness eyelid tissue containing the offending cilium and follicle are removed and the wound left unsutured. (Redrawn with permission from: Petersen-Jones SM and Crispin SM (eds) *Manual of Small Animal Ophthalmology*, Cheltenham: British Small Animal Veterinary Association Publications 1993).

corneal ulcers, particularly superficial ones, are painful and result in blepharospasm and increased lacrimation. There are a number of potential causes of corneal ulceration as listed below [6]:

- Trauma
- Chemicals – alkalis, acids, detergents
- Infection
    - bacterial (possibly following initial trauma)
    - viral infection (e.g. cats with feline herpesvirus infection)
    - fungal infection (rare)
- Tear film abnormalities (see p. 217–224)
- Cilia abnormalities
- Exposure keratopathy
    - brachycephalics with prominent globe/shallow orbit and poor lid closure
    - facial nerve paralysis. Most mesocephalic and dolichocephalic breeds can retract their globes sufficiently to result in a complete spread of tears across the cornea by the third eyelid, thus keeping the cornea healthy. Tear spreading by the third eyelids in brachycephalics is usually inadequate.
    - trigeminal nerve lesions. Reduced or absent corneal sensation invariably results in a keratitis affecting the area of cornea exposed between the eyelids.

- Corneal epithelial basement membrane dystrophy; this results in recurrent epithelial erosions/indolent ulcers
- Rupture of epithelial bullae in edematous corneas (e.g. those with endothelial dystrophy; see p. 68–69 and 133–134)
- Epithelial erosion by corneal cholesterol or calcium deposits in patients with lipid keratopathy or corneal calcific degeneration (see p. 73).

Investigation of corneal ulceration

A complete ocular examination is required and any predisposing factors, such as the eyelid abnormalities which were considered above, should be identified. Observation of the frequency of blinking and the extent of eyelid closure can be made during the initial examination. The tear film should be assessed early in the investigation and a Schirmer tear test performed before any fluid is applied to the ocular surface (see p. 14). Palpebral and corneal sensation should be assessed also allowing observation of the blink reflex. Magnification is useful when examining corneal lesions and the use of a slit-lamp biomicroscope is particularly helpful for judging the depth of ulcers.

Use of ophthalmic dyes in investigating corneal disease

Ophthalmic dyes are useful in the investigation of corneal pathology. Fluorescein is the most commonly used dye:

- Apply fluorescein from single dose vial or from paper impregnated strips
- Wash excess dye from ocular surface, particularly when tear production is low, to prevent false impression of staining
- Dye passes through full thickness epithelial defects to stain underlying stroma
- Fluorescein does not stain Descemet's membrane (useful for determining if defect extends down to Descemet's membrane)
- Dye will spread to stain the stroma beneath non-adherent epithelium (see non-healing superficial ulcers below)

Rose bengal is less commonly used in veterinary ophthalmology, it has the following features:

- Vital dye stains dead/damaged cells and mucus
- Rose bengal is quite irritating
- It can be used for staining superficial corneal epithelial damage
- It is useful for staining epithelial defects in cats due to feline herpesvirus infection (dendritic ulcers).

Laboratory investigation of corneal ulceration

Swabs for culture:

- Swab ulcers where bacterial infection is suspected or the ulcer is progressing
- Use of local anesthetic is required to allow active edge of ulcer to be sampled
- Swabs for feline herpesvirus culture must be transported to the laboratory in the appropriate transport medium.

Scrapes/smears/biopsies for histopathology:

- Sample edge of ulcer with sterile spatula after local anesthesia
- Gently smear on clean microscope slide (alcohol washed)
- Dry
- Stain – Diff Quik((Merze and Dade) provides a rapid in-house stain and is useful for both cytology and identifying the presence of bacteria. The results of a Gram's stain help in the selection of an appropriate antibiotic until culture and sensitivity results are available.
- If sending smear for indirect fluorescent antibody tests for feline herpesvirus avoid using diagnostic fluorescein as this can interfere with the test giving false positive results
- Tissue samples may be sent for polymerase chain reaction amplification to demonstrate the presence of certain infective agents (e.g. feline herpesvirus); contact the laboratories offering this service before sampling.

Management of Corneal Ulcers

Superficial uncomplicated ulcers will normally heal within a few days and topical antibiotic cover is all that is required.

Non-healing superficial ulcers (Figure 6.9) (indolent ulcers, recurrent epithelial erosions, boxer ulcers) are a specific form of ulcer that require intervention to facilitate healing. They are thought to be due to abnormalities of adherence of epithelium to the basement membrane and of the basement membrane itself [7, 8]. These ulcers have the following characteristics:

- They occur in dogs and much less commonly cats
- They are superficial and involve epithelium only
- There may or may not be a history of minor trauma
- There is little tendency to heal; can persist for months
- They are surrounded by a zone of non-adherent epithelium (fluorescein passes under this, staining the stroma beyond the apparent edge of the ulcer)

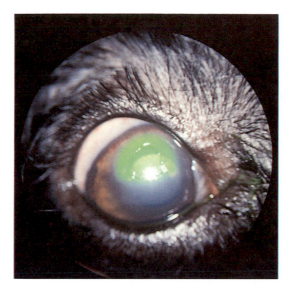

Figure 6.9 A superficial non-healing ulcer. This has been stained with fluorescein. Note the characteristic staining beyond the edge of the epithelial defect. This is due to non-adherence of the surrounding epithelium.

- There is a variable extent of accompanying corneal edema and vascularization.

Several methods of managing non-healing ulcers have been advocated. One of the most effective methods is first to remove all loose epithelium surrounding the ulcer and then to create shallow stromal wounds in a puctate or linear fashion [9, 10] (Figure 6.10). A cotton tipped swab, spatula, or scalpel blade (using a sideways brushing motion) is used to remove non-adherent epithelium, which may cover a large area of the cornea. Multiple anterior stromal punctures or linear wounds in a grid pattern are then made over the new extent of exposed stroma using a 23 gauge hypodermic needle. The needle is pressed perpendicularly onto the cornea until it just indents the surface. This procedure can be performed in most patients under topical anesthesia. If the cornea does not re-epithelialize within two weeks the procedure may be repeated.

Feline herpesvirus keratitis

Classic feline herpesvirus ulcers are superficial branching (dendritic) epithelial defects that are readily demonstrated by rose bengal staining. Less commonly a more extensive keratitis may develop characterized by a marked corneal cellular infiltrate, and in some cases may lead to serious ulceration (probably contributed to by secondary

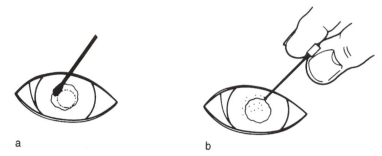

a   b

Figure 6.10 Treatment for a superficial non-healing ulcer. (a) All surrounding loose epithelium is removed using a dry swab, a spatula, or a scalpel blade. (b) A punctate keratotomy is performed using a hypodermic needle to make multiple superficial wounds into the anterior corneal stroma.

pathogens). Antiviral therapy using trifluorothymidine or idoxuridine may be effective. The efficacy of acyclovir may be improved by concurrent application of topical interferon.

Deep corneal ulcers

Deeper ulcers (Figure 6.11) may potentially lead to corneal perforation. Liquefaction of the collagen-rich corneal stroma due to the

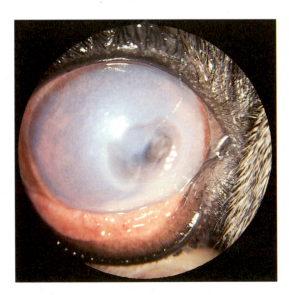

Figure 6.11 A deep ulcer in a pug. Note the red appearance of the eye and the corneal edema. The clearer center to the ulcer suggests that it deepens to the level of Descemet's membrane and is at risk of perforating.

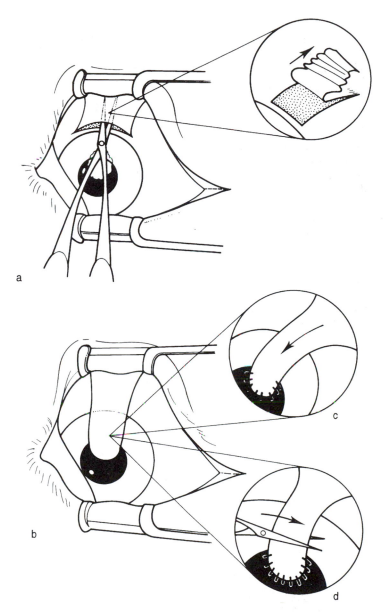

Figure 6.12   Application of a conjunctival pedicle flap for treatment of a deep corneal ulcer. (a) An initial paralimbal incision has been made and the bulbar conjunctiva is being undermined by blunt and sharp dissection with scissors. The bulbar conjunctiva is translucent, (*caption continued overleaf*)

action of proteolytic enzymes released from bacteria or neutrophils can result in devastating, rapidly progressive or melting ulcers. Swabs and scrapes should be taken to investigate possible bacterial infection. Potential corneal pathogens include coagulase positive staphylococci, β-hemolytic streptococci, *Pseudomonas aeruginosa* (notorious as a cause of melting ulcers) and other Gram-negative bacteria. For progressive or melting ulcers intensive treatment with an appropriate antibiotic should be started (e.g. for *Pseudomonas aeruginosa* infections gentamicin, tobramycin, or ciprofloxacin). For serious ulcers resulting from Gram-positive infections cephazolin has been advocated and a suitable preparation may be made by adding cephazolin for intravenous use to an artificial tear preparation to a final concentration of 33 mg ml^{-1} [11]. In most instances where corneal melting is not a problem the use of a commercial broad spectrum topical antibiotic is sufficient.

Suturing the third eyelid across the eye (preferably to the bulbar conjunctiva rather than through the upper eyelid) remains a useful mode of therapy, providing support and protection to the ulcer. Care should be taken to ensure that the sutures do not abrade the cornea. Unfortunately the cornea cannot be observed while the third eyelid is sutured across the eye, so deepening of the ulcer will not be apparent until perforation occurs. When the ulcer is deeper than approximately one-half the thickness of the cornea a conjunctival flap or pedicle graft is preferable.

A variety of conjunctival flaps have been described. These have the advantage of providing protection and support for the weakened cornea. The blood supply provided directly to the ulcer site aids in

---

scissors to be clearly visualised. Dissection is continued towards the fornix. Two divergent incisions are then made towards the fornix. Once these incisions have been made and the bulbar conjunctival pedicle has been freed from the underlying episclera, it is possible to achieve a substantial length of pedicle. A lateral canthotomy has been performed in this diagram. (b) The conjunctival pedicle graft has been advanced to overlie the recipient ulcer bed. The base of the pedicle is usually at the conjunctival fornix. It is necessary to loosen or remove the eyelid retractors to allow the pedicle graft to be advanced onto the ulcer site without undue tension. (c) The ventromedial, ventral and ventrolateral borders of the pedicle graft are sutured to the recipient ulcer bed with 7.0 or 8.0 absorbable suture. (d) One blade of a pair of scissors is slid beneath the non-adherent pedicle bridge (as shown in (c)) when the pedicle bridge is to be sectioned 4–6 weeks postoperatively. Steven's tenotomy scissors are ideal as the ends are slightly blunted, thereby reducing the risk of corneal damage if the animal moves suddenly while the pedicle bridge is cut. (Redrawn with permission from: Habin D. Conjunctival pedicle grafts. *In Practice* 1995; **17**: 61–65).

Table 6·1   Causes of glaucoma

Primary	• Goniodysgenesis
	• Primary open angle glaucoma
Secondary	• Primary lens luxation — terrier breeds, border collie
	• Uveitis, including lens-induced uveitis
	• Neoplasia
	• Neovascular tissue overlying the pectinate ligament — secondary to retinal detachment, neoplasia or uveitis
	• Intraocular hemorrhage
	• Intumescence (swelling) of a cataractous lens
	• Pigmentary glaucoma (Cairn terriers)
	• Vitreous prolapse after surgical lens extraction

corneal healing and has an antibacterial and antiprotease action which can help control bacterial infection and corneal liquefaction. The pedicle flap (Figure 6.12) is useful for the treatment of deep ulcers, descemetoceles and even ulcers that have perforated [12, 13].

GLAUCOMA

Glaucoma is a pathological increase in intraocular pressure (IOP) which causes optic nerve head and retinal damage and subsequent blindness. When the IOP increases rapidly, pain is often a major presenting sign. The normal IOP is 15 to 25 mmHg. Measurement of IOP is considered on p. 18–20 and 21–22.

Glaucoma arises as a result of impaired drainage of aqueous humor from the eye. The defect in the drainage pathway may be at the pupil or the iridocorneal angle. Glaucoma may be primary, or secondary to other ocular disease (Table 6.1). Goniodysgenesis is the commonest cause of primary glaucoma and constitutes the presence of a congenitally abnormal sheet of tissue at the site of the pectinate ligament, with associated narrowing of the entrance to the ciliary cleft [14, 15]. Examination of the iridocorneal drainage angle is described on p. 22.

Clinical signs of glaucoma

When considering clinical signs, glaucoma may be divided into acute and chronic forms [16].

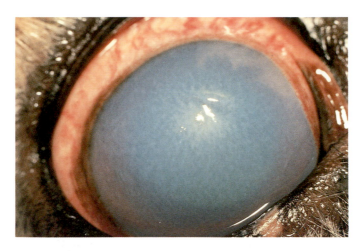

Figure 6.13   Corneal edema in a Dandie Dinmont terrier with primary glaucoma due to goniodysgenesis. Rupture of a corneal bulla has resulted in a small corneal ulcer.

Acute glaucoma (also see pages 114–116)

Acute onset cases tend to present with signs of a painful eye, i.e. blepharospasm, epiphora, and head-shyness. The pain may be so severe as to cause yelping, lethargy, and anorexia. Blindness may develop rapidly and can become irreversible after 24 to 48 hr. Corneal edema is often seen due to fluid from the aqueous not being cleared from the cornea (Figure 6.13). Episcleral congestion is a major presenting sign in both acute and chronic glaucoma cases (Figure 6.14). It may also be present in cases of episcleritis, uveitis, and orbital disease, from which glaucoma must be differentiated.

Increased IOP leads to paralysis of the iris sphincter muscle and the pupil tends to become mid-dilated and poorly mobile. Acute onset glaucoma most commonly results from goniodysgenesis, lens luxation, or uveitis.

Chronic glaucoma (also see pages 139–140)

With chronicity the signs of pain may become less obvious, but the capacity for glaucoma to cause discomfort should never be underestimated.

Chronic cases may exhibit some or all of the signs associated with acute disease, but often to a lesser degree. In addition, the globe enlarges (hydrophthalmos) and this may lead to lens subluxation or luxation, breaks in Descemet's membrane which are seen as gray streaks in the cornea (Figure 6.15) and staphyloma formation (blue

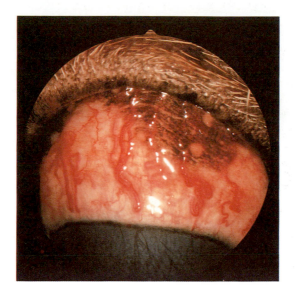

Figure 6.14 Episcleral vascular congestion in a Labrador retriever with glaucoma.

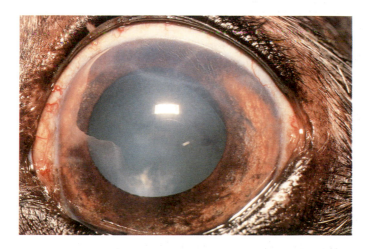

Figure 6.15 Breaks in Descemet's membrane in the enlarged globe of a Staffordshire bull terrier with chronic primary glaucoma. The lesions are seen as gray lines in the dorsal cornea.

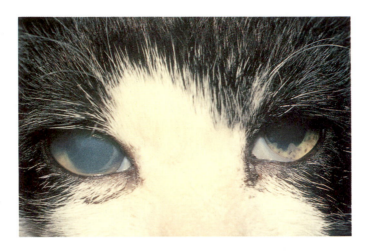

Figure 6.16   Chronic glaucoma with globe enlargement in the right eye of a domestic cat with bilateral anterior uveitis. The left eye exhibits keratic precipitates on the ventral corneal endothelium.

swelling at the equator of the globe). The cornea may become vascularized and pigmented, and cataract or intraocular hemorrhage may occur. Fundus changes include optic disc cupping, seen as a posterior bowing of the optic nerve head, and retinal degeneration.

Primary open angle glaucoma, glaucoma secondary to neoplasia, and some cases resulting from uveitis are most likely to present as insidious, chronic disease. Cats commonly present with chronic glaucoma secondary to low-grade uveitis (Figure 6.16).

Management

Therapy may be medical or surgical. Glaucoma often carries a guarded outlook for vision and aggressive therapy is usually required if vision is to be preserved.

Medical treatment (also see pages 35–37)

Osmotic diuretics

Mannitol 10 to 20% solution, 1 to 2 g/kg given iv over 20 min may be used for rapid reduction of IOP. Care should be taken with its use in elderly or sick patients.

Carbonic anhydrase inhibitors

These are the mainstay of medical therapy and act to inhibit aqueous production [17]. Various drugs are available (Table 6.2). Adverse

Table 6·2   Carbonic anhydrase inhibitors

Drug	Dosage
Dorzolamide hydrochloride	2% solution TID topically
Ethoxzolamide	4 to 7.5 mg/kg BID to TID per os
Methazolamide	5 to 10 mg/kg BID to TID per os
Dichlorphenamide	5 to 10 mg/kg BID to TID per os
Acetazolamide	10 to 25 mg/kg BID per os

BID = twice daily; TID = three times daily.

effects to systemic therapy include diuresis, gastrointestinal disturbances, hypokalemia, and metabolic acidosis. Potassium supplements should be given with long-term oral treatment. Topical use of carbonic anhydrase inhibitors avoids systemic side effects.

β-adrenergic blockers

β-blockers applied topically result in reduced aqueous production. They can be a useful adjunct to therapy, but generally their effect is insufficient to be used alone. Timolol maleate and metipranolol applied twice to three times daily are the most commonly used agents.

Miotics

Where the drainage apparatus is still open, topical miotics such as pilocarpine and demecarium bromide cause a reduction in IOP. Their use is questionable when the ciliary cleft is blocked or covered by abnormal tissue, as is true of most small animal glaucoma cases.

Surgical treatment

Surgery may be directed at decreasing the production of aqueous or increasing its outflow.

Cyclodestructive techniques

Partial destruction of the ciliary body can be achieved using cryotherapy [18], laser therapy [19], or chemical ablation with intravitreal gentamicin [20]. Of these, laser therapy is the technique of choice.

Drainage procedures

Scleral trephination combined with peripheral iridectomy is a simple method of temporarily increasing aqueous outflow [21]. Drainage implants of various types are currently preferred as they reduce the risk of failure due to scar tissue formation which prevents reabsorption of aqueous [22, 23].

Enucleation or evisceration with intraocular prosthesis

Some blind, painful, glaucomatous eyes cannot be successfully managed by the techniques outlined above. In these cases, enucleation or evisceration with insertion of a silicone sphere may be the best option available.

ACUTE ANTERIOR UVEITIS

Anterior uveitis constitutes inflammation of the iris and the ciliary body [24–26]. Acute uveitis can cause intense ocular pain, mainly as a result of ciliary and iris muscle spasm. Chronic uveitis is dealt with on p. 134–139.

Causes of anterior uveitis include infection (Table 6.3), trauma (Figure 6.17), corneal insult, intraocular neoplasia, and immune-mediated disease (including lens-induced uveitis [27] due to lens trauma or cataract). Less commonly it may be associated with granulomatous meningoencephalitis, hyperviscosity syndrome, or hypertension.

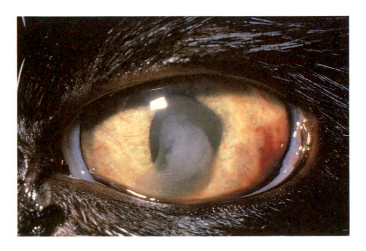

Figure 6.17　Acute traumatic uveitis in the left eye of a cat. A limbal wound has resulted in hemorrhage, iris swelling, posterior synechia formation with consequent pupil distortion, and the development of a fibrin clot within the aqueous.

Table 6·3   Infectious causes of uveitis

Dog		Cat	

Viral	Canine adenovirus
	Canine distemper
	Rabies
		Viral	Feline infectious peritonitis
			  virus
			Feline leukemia virus
			Feline immunosuppressive
			  virus

Bacterial	Leptospirosis
	Borreliosis (Lyme disease)
	Brucellosis
	Miscellaneous infections
	  (pyometra, tooth root abscess
	  etc.)
		Bacterial	Tuberculosis
			Miscellaneous infections

Fungal	Coccidioidomycosis Blastomycosis Histoplasmosis Cryptococcosis	Fungal	Cryptococcosis Histoplasmosis Blastomycosis Coccidioidomycosis
Protozoal	Toxoplasmosis Leishmaniasis	Protozoal	Toxoplasmosis

Parasitic	Toxocariasis
	Dirofilariasis
	Angiostrongylus
	Migrating fly larvae
	  (ophthalmomyiasis
	  internal)
		Parasitic	Migrating fly larvae
			  (ophthalmomyiasis
			  internal)

Rickettsial	Ehrlichiosis Rocky Mountain Spotted Fever		
Algal	Protothecosis		

Clinical signs

Acute anterior uveitis may cause combinations of the following signs [28]:

- Evidence of pain – blepharospasm, enophthalmos, photophobia, lacrimation, protrusion of third eyelid
- Episcleral and conjunctival congestion (Figure 6.18)
- Miosis (constricted pupil)
- Aqueous flare (protein) and cells in the anterior chamber (Figure 6.18)
- Keratic precipitates on the corneal endothelium, especially ventrally (Figure 6.16)
- Hypopyon (white blood cells in the anterior chamber) (Figure 6.19)

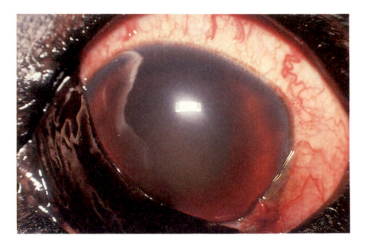

Figure 6.18   Marked aqueous flare in a 10 year old Labrador retriever with anterior uveitis secondary to intraocular lymphosarcoma. Moderate episcleral congestion is also present.

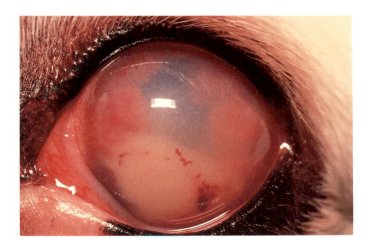

Figure 6.19   Hypopyon, intraocular hemorrhage, intense iris congestion, and corneal edema in the eye of a cat with acute anterior uveitis.

- Hyphema (red blood cells in the anterior chamber) (Figure 6.20)
- Corneal edema (Figure 6.19)
- Deep corneal vascularization
- Iris swelling and congestion (Figure 6.19)
- Synechiae formation (adhesions between iris and lens or cornea) (Figure 6.17)

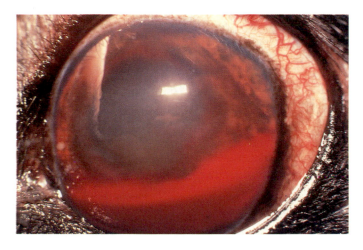

Figure 6.20   Hyphema in the left eye of a crossbred dog with acute anterior uveitis.

- Iris bombé (360° posterior synechiae with resultant bowing forward of the iris and glaucoma)
- Lowered intraocular pressure.

Diagnosis

The diagnosis of anterior uveitis depends upon assessment of signalment and history (especially important as associated systemic disease may be present), and is particularly reliant upon a careful ophthalmic examination. Some signs of acute uveitis, such as aqueous flare and keratic precipitates, may be subtle and are best detected in a darkened room using a focal light source and good magnification, e.g. a slit-lamp biomicroscope. The use of tonometry is important in the assessment of a suspected case of anterior uveitis as lowered IOP may be an early indicator of the disease. Diagnosis of the cause of uveitis may involve extensive laboratory work-up and thorough investigation of the case for evidence of systemic disease [29–31].

Numerous diseases may mimic the signs of anterior uveitis, especially where redness of the ocular coats is a feature [32]. Most notably these include glaucoma, episcleritis, keratitis, conjunctivitis and retrobulbar cellulitis. Miosis, enophthalmos and conjunctival vascular injection are features common to both uveitis and Horner's syndrome (see p. 59–60).

Management

The main aims are to remove any underlying cause, control inflammation and to relieve pain.

Anti-inflammatory therapy [33]

Corticosteroids may be used topically and systemically in the treatment of anterior uveitis. Prednisolone acetate applied topically provides good intraocular penetration.

Non-steroidal anti-inflammatory drugs (NSAID) may also be used systemically and topically for treatment of uveitis. Topical treatment is most useful before and after intraocular surgery. Some of the drugs available for systemic use are indicated in Table 6.4 (availability and data sheet details vary between countries). In severe cases, anti-inflammatory therapy may be supplemented with the use of immunosuppressive agents. The drug most commonly employed is azathioprine (2 mg/kg on alternate days).

Mydriatic cycloplegics

Dilating the pupil reduces the likelihood of synechia formation and decreasing iris and ciliary muscle spasm relieves pain. Topical 1% atropine is used four times daily initially. Where severe miosis or iris bombé are present, 10% phenylephrine may be used for its additive action. Mid-dilation is desirable as maximal dilation may compromise aqueous drainage.

When managing uveitis cases, the dosage of treatment is gradually reduced over a period of several weeks or months in order to reduce

Table 6·4   Anti-inflammatory drugs

	Drugs	Dosage
Corticosteroids		
Topical	Prednisolone acetate 1%	4 to 6 times daily initially (more
	Dexamethasone 0.1%	often) in severe cases)
Systemic	Prednisolone	0.5 to 1 mg/kg/day initially (or
	Methylprednisolone	higher doses in severe or
		autoimmune cases)
Non-steroidals		
Topical	Flurbiprofen 0.03%	Various human data sheet dosage
	Diclofenac sodium 0.1%	schedules for perioperative use
	Suprofen 1%	
Systemic – dogs	Carprophen	2 to 4 mg/kg/day initially
	Meloxicam	0.2 mg/kg once daily initially
	Flunixin meglumine	0.25 to 0.5 mg/kg sid 3 days
Systemic – cats	Ketoprofen	1mg/kg once daily 5 days
	Phenylbutazone	5 to 10 mg/kg twice daily

the likelihood of relapse. Careful monitoring, including regular measurement of the intraocular pressure, is required during this period.

LENS LUXATION

Dislocation of the lens may occur as a primary or a secondary event.

Primary lens luxation

Primary lens luxation is seen most commonly in middle-aged terrier breeds and the border collie [34, 35]. A congenital abnormality of the lens zonule leads to a progressive breakdown of zonules resulting in subluxation and subsequent luxation of the lens.

Pain is often a major presenting feature of anterior lens luxation. The lens may be visible in the anterior chamber and is most easily recognized by the presence of a bright, refractile ring which represents the lens equator (Figure 6.21). Sub-central corneal edema may result from the luxated lens contacting the cornea. Prior to complete luxation, the unsupported iris may be seen to tremble (iridodonesis) and prolapsed vitreous may be seen as grayish strands in the anterior chamber.

Secondary glaucoma commonly results from lens luxation in dogs due to blockage of the pupil by the lens or vitreous, or as a result of

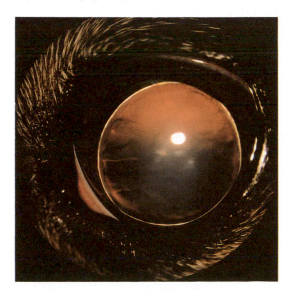

Figure 6.21   Primary lens luxation in a Parson Jack Russell terrier. The lens is positioned in the anterior chamber and can be recognized by the refractile ring of the lens equator.

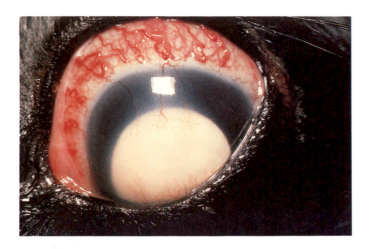

Figure 6.22   Secondary lens luxation in a dog with glaucoma and globe enlargement. The lens is within the anterior chamber and has become cataractous.

obstruction of the drainage angle by vitreous. Blindness may rapidly ensue due to optic nerve damage. Glaucoma secondary to anterior lens luxation is uncommon in cats, probably due to the depth of the feline anterior chamber.

Treatment involves rapidly reducing the intraocular pressure (see p. 186) followed by intracapsular lens extraction.

Secondary lens luxation

The lens may dislocate due to damage to the zonular attachments resulting from antecedent ocular disease. The major cause is glaucoma inducing enlargement of the globe and stretching of the zonular fibers (Figure 6.22). However, lens luxation may also result from uveitis [36] and severe trauma. Where lens luxation is secondary to other ocular disease, lens extraction is less likely to be indicated. Efforts should first be directed towards control of the underlying problem before considering surgical intervention.

REFERENCES

1. Mould JRB. Conditions of the orbit and globe. In: Petersen-Jones SM & Crispin SM (eds) *Manual of Small Animal Ophthalmology*, Cheltenham: BSAVA Publications 1993; 49–50.
2. McCalla TL and Moore CP. Exophthalmos in dogs and cats – part II. *Comp. Cont. Educ. Pract. Vet.* 1989; **11**: 911–26.
3. Petersen-Jones SM. Conditions of the eyelid and nictitating membrane.

In: Petersen-Jones SM & Crispin SM (eds) *Manual of Small Animal Ophthalmology*, Cheltenham: BSAVA Publications 1993; 70–2.

4. Johnson BW, Gerding PA, McLaughlin SA, Helper LC, Szajerski ME and Cormany KA. Nonsurgical correction of entropion in Shar Pei puppies. *Vet Med* 1988; **83**: 482–3.

5. Stades FC. A new method for surgical correction of upper eyelid trichiasis-entropion: operation method. *J. Am. Anim. Hosp. Ass.* 1987; **23**: 603–10.

6. Nasisse MP. Canine ulcerative keratitis. *Comp. Cont. Educ. Pract. Vet.* 1985; **7**: 686–701.

7. Gelatt KN and Samuelson DA. Recurrent corneal erosions and epithelial dystrophy in the boxer dog. *J. Am. Anim. Hosp. Ass.* 1982; **18**: 453–60.

8. Kirschner SE, Niyo Y and Betts DM. Idiopathic persistent corneal erosions: clinical and pathological findings in 18 dogs. *J. Am. Anim. Hosp. Ass.* 1989; **25**: 84–90.

9. Champagne ES and Munger RJ. Multiple punctate keratotomy for the treatment of recurrent epithelial erosions in dogs. *J. Am. Anim. Hosp. Ass.* 1992; **28**: 213–6.

10. Morgan RV and Abrams KL. A comparison of six different therapies for persistent corneal erosions in dogs and cats. *Prog. Vet. Comp. Ophthalmol.* 1994; **4**: 38–43.

11. Baum J. Therapy for ocular bacterial infection. *Trans. Ophthalmol. Soc. UK* 1986; **105**: 69–77.

12. Håkanson N and Merideth RE. Conjunctival pedicle grafting in the treatment of corneal ulcers in the dog and cat. *J. Am. Anim. Hosp. Ass.* 1987; **23**: 641–8.

13. Håkanson N, Lorimer D and Meredith RE. Further comments on the conjunctival pedicle grafting in the treatment of corneal ulcers in the dog and cat. *J. Am. Anim. Hosp. Ass.* 1988; **24**: 602–5.

14. Brooks DE. Glaucoma in the dog and cat. *Vet. Clin. North. Am. (Small Anim. Pract.)* 1990; **20**: 775–97.

15. Renwick PW. Glaucoma. In: Petersen-Jones SM & Crispin SM (eds) *Manual of Small Animal Ophthalmology*, Cheltenham: BSAVA Publications 1993; 193–212.

16. Barnett KC. Glaucoma. In: Barnett KC (ed) *A Colour Atlas of Veterinary Ophthalmology*, London: Wolfe Publishing 1990: 70–4.

17. Regnier A and Toutain PL. Ocular pharmacology and therapeutic modalities: antiglaucomatous drugs In: Gelatt KN (ed) *Veterinary Ophthalmology*, 2nd edn. Philadelphia: Lea & Febiger 1991: 175–81.

18. Roberts SM, Severin GA and Lavach JD. Cyclocryotherapy – Part I. Evaluation of a liquid nitrogen system. *J. Am. Anim. Hosp. Ass.* 1984; **20**: 823–7.

19. Nasisse MP, Davidson MG and English RV. Treatment of glaucoma by use of transscleral neodymium;yttrium aluminium garnet laser cyclocoagulation in dogs. *J. Am. Vet. Med. Ass.* 1990; **197**: 350–4.

20. Moller I, Cook CS, Peiffer RL, Nasisse MP and Harling DEl. Indications for and complications of pharmacological ablation of the ciliary body for the treatment of chronic glaucoma in the dog. *J. Am. Anim. Hosp. Ass.* 1986; **22**: 319–26.

21. Bedford PGC. The surgical treatment of canine glaucoma. *J. Small Anim. Pract.* 1977; **18**: 713–30.
22. Bedford PGC. A clinical evaluation of a one-piece drainage system in the treatment of canine glaucoma. *J. Small Anim. Pract.* 1989; **30**: 68–75.
23. Gelatt KN, Brooks DE, Miller TR, Smiht PJ, Sapienza JS and Pellicane CP. Issues in ophthalmic therapy: The development of anterior chamber shunts for the clinical management of canine glaucomas. *Prog. Vet. Comp. Ophthalmol.* 1992; **2**: 59–64.
24. Håkanson N and Forrester SD. Uveitis in the dog and cat. *Vet. Clin. North. Am. (Small Anim. Pract.)* 1990; **20**: 715–35.
25. Collins BK and Moore CP. Canine anterior uvea. In: Gelatt KN (ed) *Veterinary Ophthalmology*, 2nd edn. Philadelphia: Lea & Febiger 1991: 357–91.
26. Crispin SM. The uveal tract. In: Petersen-Jones SM & Crispin SM (eds) *Manual of Small Animal Ophthalmology*, Cheltenham: BSAVA Publications 1993; 173–91.
27. van der Woerdt A, Nasisse MP and Davidson MG. Lens-induced uveitis in dogs: 151 cases (1985–1990). *J. Am. Vet. Med. Ass.* 1992; **201**: 921–6.
28. Barnett KC. The Iris. In: Barnett KC (ed) *A Colour Atlas of Veterinary Ophthalmology*, London: Wolfe Publishing 1990: 55–69.
29. Davidson MG, Nasisse MP, English RV, Wilcock BP and Jamieson VE. Feline anterior uveitis: A study of 53 cases. *J. Am. Anim. Hosp. Ass.* 1991; **27**: 77–83.
30. Hopper CD and Crispin S. Differential diagnosis of uveitis in cats. *In Pract.* 1992; **14**: 289–97.
31. Lappin MR, Marks A, Greene CE, Collins JK, Carman J, Reif SJ and Powell CC. Serologic prevalence of selected infectious diseases in cats with uveitis. *J. Am. Vet. Med. Ass.* 1992; **201**: 1005–9.
32. Petersen-Jones SM. Differential diagnosis of the 'red eye' in small animals. *In Pract.* 1993; **15**: 55–64.
33. Regneir A and Toutain PL. Ocular pharmacology and therapeutic modalities: anti-inflammatory drugs. In: Gelatt KN (ed) *Veterinary Ophthalmology*, 2nd edn. Philadelphia: Lea & Febiger 1991: 171–5.
34. Curtis R. Lens luxation in the dog and cat. *Vet. Clin. North. Am. (Small Anim. Pract.)* 1990; **20**: 755–73.
35. Foster SJ, Curtis R and Barnett KC. Primary lens luxation in the Border Collie. *J. Small Anim. Pract.* 1986; **27**: 1–6.
36. Olivero DK, Riis RC, Dutton AG, Murphy CJ, Nasisse MP and Davidson MG. Feline lens displacement: A retrospective analysis of 345 cases. *Prog. Vet. Comp. Ophthalmol.* 1991; **1**: 239–44.

7

Ocular Discharge

Richard I E Smith, Robin G Stanley, Jeffrey S Smith and Simon M Petersen-Jones

This chapter starts with a description of the normal preocular tear film and the techniques used to assess it. Conditions which present with ocular discharge as the primary sign are then considered under the following three sections:

- Abnormal ocular discharges in the presence of normal or increased aqueous tear production as measured by the Schirmer tear test
- Overflow of normal tears and increased tear production
- Reduced tear production (dry eye) and altered tear mucus or lipid

THE NORMAL PREOCULAR TEAR FILM

The normal ocular surface secretion is the tear film which is a complex liquid that covers the exposed cornea and conjunctiva and is essential for maintaining a normal ocular surface [1]. The tear film is made up of three different layers secreted by glandular components of the lacrimal system and is distributed over the surface of the eye by the action of the eyelids and drained by a pumping action of the eyelids through the puncta into the nasolacrimal drainage system. The outermost layer of the tear film is a lipid layer secreted primarily by modified sebaceous glands, the meibomian glands, which are situated within the eyelids (Figure 7.1). These glands open onto the eyelid margin and their secretion has the primary function of stabilizing the tear film, reducing evaporation, lubricating lid movement over the ocular surface, and preventing contamination of the ocular surface by the more polar lipids of the skin. The middle, or aqueous layer of the tear film, is produced by the lacrimal gland, and also the gland of the third eyelid. Tear film mucins form the majority of the inner layer of the tear film which acts to bind the outer layers to the surface microvilli of the conjunctival and corneal epithelial cells. The mucus layer consists of two parts; an innermost glycocalyx secreted by the epithelial cells themselves, and a hydrated glycoprotein mucinous layer secreted by the unicellular conjunctival goblet cells which are present at greatest density in the conjunctival fornix [2] (Figure

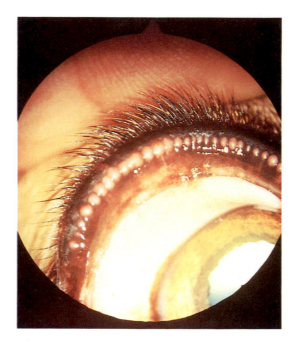

Figure 7.1   Row of meibomian glands discharging white lipid onto eyelid margin in a dog.

7.2). Dogs and cats may also produce varying quantities of mucus from the gland of the third eyelid.

The tear film physiology is complex and fascinating:

- The flushing action of the tears helps to trap and remove debris from the ocular surfaces.
- The action of non-specific antibacterial substances such as lysozyme, betalysin, and lactoferrin, combined with specific protective immunoglobulins help protect the ocular surface from infection.
- The tear film also provides a pathway for white blood cells from the limbal and conjunctival circulation to reach the cornea in cases of ocular surface disease.
- Oxygen and nutrients are supplied to the avascular cornea via the tear film and waste products, including desquamated epithelial cells are removed.

Alterations in the tear film may be caused by local and/or systemic problems and may have a deleterious effect on the ocular surface.

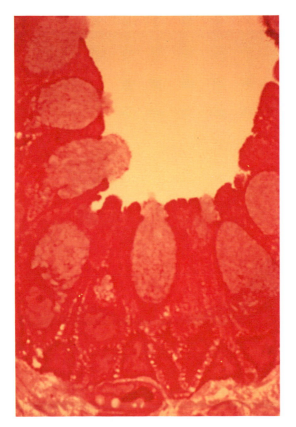

Figure 7.2   Goblet cells in conjunctival fornix discharging mucus.

Examination of the tear film

A visual assessment of the tear film forms part of every ophthalmic examination. The reflection of the examining light from the cornea should be clean and even. Close examination should reveal a tear meniscus between the lower eyelid margin and corneal surface. At the medial canthus there is a slightly deeper accumulation of tears (the medial canthal lake) and often at this site there is an accumulation of mucus.

The Schirmer tear test is used to measure aqueous tear production (Figure 7.3). The test is performed by placing standardized strips of absorbent paper between the corneal surface and the lower eyelid to measure the reflex tears produced in 1 min. In most normal dogs there is over 15 mm of wetting and in cats more than 10 mm. This test should be performed early in the examination before adding any fluid

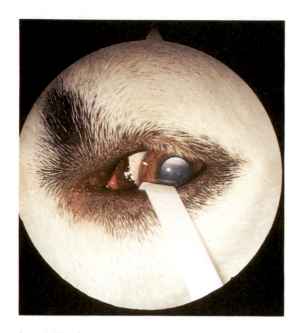

Figure 7.3   Schirmer filter paper testing aqueous tear production in a dog.

to the eye or unduly manipulating the eye. Specialized methods can be used to assess the lipid and mucus phases of the tear film. These are considered further on p. 224.

The normal conjunctiva

The conjunctiva is a vascularized mucous membrane which extends from the lid margin to the limbus. As such, it covers the inner surface of the eyelids, turning at the fornix to overly the globe and cover both surfaces of the third eyelid. It contains the unicellular mucus-secreting goblet cells and plays a role in the ocular immune system through specialized lymphoid aggregates called conjunctival-associated lymphoid tissue (CALT). Limbal antigen presenting cells, the Langerhan's cells, also play a role with CALT. Microorganisms are present in the conjunctival sac of many normal animals, but usually at low numbers. Gram-positive bacteria are the commonest microorganisms found in the dog and cat conjunctival sac, although Gram-negative organisms can be isolated at a lower frequency [3, 4].

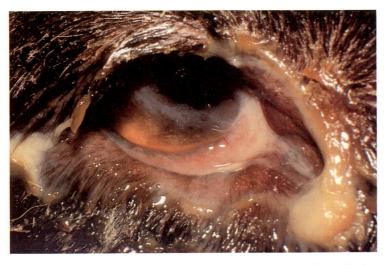

Figure 7.4 A Pointer dog with a copious chronic mucopurulent discharge. The cornea is not involved but the conjunctiva shows mild chemosis suggesting that this is a conjunctivitis. The discharges themselves may irritate the surrounding skin causing a moist dermatitis. To find the cause of the discharge a detailed ocular examination should be performed. Pay particular attention to the history. Remember to examine the adjacent orbital structures such as teeth and sinuses.

ABNORMAL OCULAR DISCHARGE IN THE PRESENCE OF NORMAL TEAR PRODUCTION

'Local' problems which alter tear secretions include inflammation of the eyelids, conjunctiva, cornea, and nasolacrimal system, and intra-ocular disease. Orbital and paranasal sinus lesions may occasionally drain through the conjunctiva causing an abnormal secretion from the eye (Figure 7.4).

Conjunctival abnormalities

Signs of inflammation of the conjunctiva are the same as those of other tissues; vascular dilation (hyperemia), tissue edema (chemosis), and exudation. The exudate results from vascular stasis, cellular exudation, and leakage of fluid containing fibrin and immunoglobulins from the involved blood vessels. According to its main component the exudate may be described as serous, mucoid, purulent, or any combination, such as mucopurulent. Conditions may be acute, subacute, or chronic. Additional changes can include conjunctival hemorrhage, emphysema (sinus fractures), follicle formation (the conjunctiva is rich in lymphoid tissue), abnormal swelling and, if the condition causes puritus, alopecia and excoriation of the eyelids and surrounding skin.

Conjunctival disease in dogs

There are many possible causes of conjunctivitis in dogs some of which are included in Table 7.1.

Infectious canine conjunctivitis

Conjunctivitis is characterized by irritation, hyperemia, and a mucopurulent discharge. Bacterial conjunctivitis may result either from overgrowth of bacteria normally found in the conjunctival sac or from contamination from the surroundings. Gram-positive bacteria are most commonly involved and there is often a predisposing factor which allows the bacteria to infect the tissue despite the actions of the

Table 7·1   Potential causes of ocular discharges

	Dog	Cat
Bacterial	Streptococci, staphylococci, pseudomonas	Streptococci, staphylococci, pseudomonas, mycoplasma,
Chlamydia	–	Chlamydial conjunctivitis
Fungal	Candida, aspergillus	Candida, aspergillus, curvilaria
Viral	Distemper, adenovirus	Feline herpesvirus (FHV), calcivirus (FCV), reovirus (RRI)
Allergic	Atopy, follicular conjunctivitis, food allergy	Atopy, food allergy
Toxic or chemical	Detergents, acids, alkalis	Detergents, acids, alkalis
Foreign bodies	Grass awns, thorns, etc.	Grass awns, thorns, etc.
Auto-immune diseases	Pemphigus group, chronic superficial keratitis, plasmacytic infiltration of the third eyelid	Pemphigus group, eosinophillic keratoconjunctivitis
Lid abnormalities	Entropion, ectropion, coloboma, cicatrical deformity, lash disorders	Entropion, ectropion, coloboma, cicatrical deformity, lash disorders
Tear film deficiency (KCS)	KCS, qualitative tear film disorders	KCS (less common)
Trauma	Blunt trauma, plant material, fights, motor vehicle accidents	Blunt trauma, fights, motor vehicle accidents
Intraocular disease	Glaucoma, anterior uveitis	Glaucoma, anterior uveitis
Extension from sinus/ orbit	Fungal, neoplasia	Fungal, neoplasia

ocular surface defense mechanisms. The investigation of a dog with conjunctivitis should include an examination for any such predisposing factors, for example, a Schirmer tear test and examining the fornix and under the third eyelid for foreign bodies such as grass awns. Most cases of conjunctivitis are self-limiting, although treatment with broad spectrum antibiotics may expedite resolution. A few cases become chronic, these should be re-examined for predisposing factors and sampled for bacterial culture and antibiotic sensitivity testing. Rickettsial diseases are seen in some parts of the world and subconjunctival petechial hemorrhages may be a feature, for example with Ehrlichiosis and Rocky Mountain spotted fever. Viral diseases such as canine distemper and canine adenoviruses may cause chemosis and seromucoid to mucopurulent discharges. Distemper can also cause a reduced tear production. Fungal conjunctivitis is not common. In Asia parasitic conjunctivitis caused by *Thelazia spp.* has been reported [5].

Hypersensitivity and immune-mediated canine conjunctival disease

Plasmacytic conjunctivitis is a chronic, probably immune-mediated, inflammatory condition of the exposed areas of the third eyelid conjunctiva. It may be accompanied by a seromucoid discharge. It is most prevalent in the German shepherd dog and may occur in conjunction with pannus (see p. 70–71 and 131). In dogs affected with the pemphigus group of diseases eyelid margin lesions are accompanied by a mucopurulent conjunctivitis. Dogs with atopy may present with epiphora and mild signs of conjunctival inflammation. Atopy is a type I hypersensitivity reaction and is initiated by inhalation of pollens, house dust, and other allergens. Follicular conjunctivitis, seen as hypertrophied lymphoid follicles scattered on the surface of the nictitans and the conjunctival fornices, occurs with chronic antigenic stimulation and is associated with seromucoid discharge [6].

Canine conjunctival neoplasia and proliferation

Squamous cell carcinoma may be seen primarily in the conjunctiva or as an extension from the eyelids. Rarely, fibrosarcoma, papilloma, lipoma, adenoma, histiocytoma, hemangioma, hemangiosarcoma, and mast cell tumors occur [7]. An inflammatory mass that can develop in the perilimbal conjunctiva is nodular granulomatous episclerokeratitis [8].

Conjunctival disease in cats

Infective feline conjunctivitis

In the cat viral conjunctivitis is common, especially in younger animals, it may be bilateral or unilateral and may produce a chronic

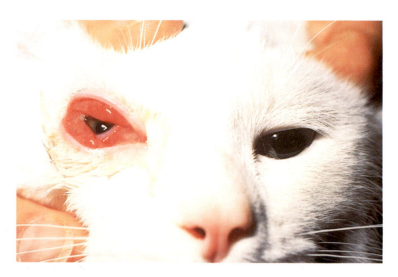

Figure 7.5 Kitten with a unilateral conjunctivitis caused by FHV-1 demonstrating hyperemia, chemosis, and a seromucoid discharge.

carrier state. Feline herpesvirus 1 (FHV 1) is a common cause of upper respiratory tract and ocular surface infection, typically in young cats. Sneezing, accompanied by nasal discharge and seromucoid to mucopurulent ocular discharges typify the early stages (Figure 7.5). There is bilateral conjunctivitis and chemosis, and in severe cases sloughing of the conjunctival epithelium may occur with resultant symblepharon formation [9] and there may also be corneal involvement. Secondary bacterial infection may complicate the picture. Chronic carrier states are possible, with recrudescence occurring during periods of stress. Calicivirus and reovirus may also produce respiratory and conjunctival disease. In the latter cases the discharge is mainly serous and there is little chemosis.

Chlamydia psittaci is another common pathogen of cats which primarily causes a conjunctivitis without respiratory infection. The condition often affects one eye first followed by the second eye a few days later [10]. There is chemosis and a copious serous discharge which may become mucopurulent with chronicity. Conjunctival lymphoid follicles may also be a feature of chronic disease (Figure 7.6). Feline pneumonitis caused by *Mycoplasma felis* and *Mycoplasma gatae* may result in epiphora, conjunctival follicle proliferation, chemosis, and a pseudomembrane.

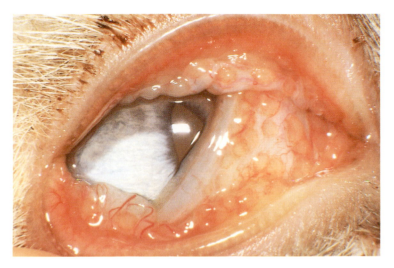

Figure 7.6 Cat with follicular conjunctivitis caused by chronic *Chlamydia psittaci* infection.

Hypersensitivity and immune-mediated feline conjunctival disease

Eosinophilic keratoconjunctivitis is a disease peculiar to cats that probably has an immune-mediated basis. The condition is characterized by a proliferative lesion affecting the conjunctiva and/or cornea and an adherent, whitish flocular surface discharge [11].

Feline conjunctival masses and neoplasms

Neoplasia reported involving the feline conjunctiva includes squamous cell carcinoma, lymphoma, and melanoma.

Investigation of conjunctival disease

Diagnosis of conjunctivitis is made from the history, clinical ocular examination and the general physical examination. To support the clinical diagnosis laboratory specimens of conjunctival cells and/or tissues are readily collected.

Samples for culture

Bacteriological investigation of dogs with severe conjunctivitis or chronic conjunctivitis that does not respond to initial treatment should be undertaken. Cats are most frequently swabbed for viral or chlamydial isolation. The appropriate transport medium should be used; for example, swabs for virus or chlamydial isolation require a

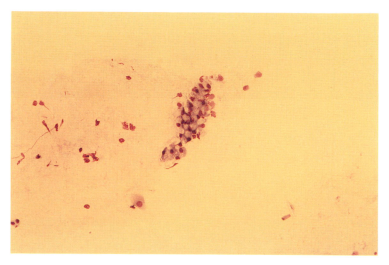

Figure 7.7   Conjunctival cytology smear stained with Diff Quik (Merze & Dade) showing conjunctival epithelial cells, goblet cells, and stained mucus.

specific transport medium. If in doubt contact the laboratory prior to sampling. When sampling for bacteriology avoid contacting the eyelid skin or eyelid margin as these sites have a different bacterial flora to the conjunctival sac and, if possible, avoid the use of topical anesthetics which may have some antibacterial action. Premoistening the swab with sterile saline is reported to improve isolation rate. It is useful, when trying to assess the significance of the results, to find out from the laboratory how heavy the bacterial growth was.

Conjunctival smears

Investigation of the conjunctival surface cytology by collecting surface smears or scrapes and staining with a Romanowski type stain and Gram's stain can be very useful (Figures 7.7 and 7.8). It is advisable first to clean the discharges from the eye using a sterile eye wash solution. Topical anesthesia can be used if required. A sterile swab, or preferably a cytology brush may be used to collect surface cells. The collected material is transferred onto a clean glass slide for cytology. Alternatively a spatula (Kimura spatula, Storz Instrument Co, St Louis) or small surgical blade are very easy to use and will collect more cells. Several slides should be made if different stains are to be used. Diff Quik (Merze and Dade) is a quick in-house Romanowski type stain which is useful for cytology. Gram's stain is used when bacterial involvement is suspected. Table 7.2 gives clinicians useful

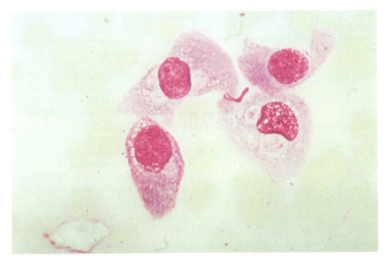

Figure 7.8 shows a smear stained with Diff Quik (Merze & Dade) from the conjunctiva of the dog shown in Figure 7.4. Note the intracytoplasmic inclusion bodies.

information to help interpret conjunctival cytology findings in dogs and cats [12]. Conjunctival smears may also be sent for immunofluorescent antibody tests, e.g. immunofluorescent antibody staining to detect canine distemper virus [13], feline herpesvirus, and *Chlamydia psittaci* [14]. Always check with the laboratory offering the service to find what they require for these tests for optimum results.

Conjunctival biopsies

Biopsies may be taken when more detailed histopathological information is required. Following repeated application of a topical anesthetic over the period a few minutes, small conjunctival biopsies may be taken. Fine forceps and sharp iris scissors can be used, taking care not to crush the tissues. It is useful to place the sample conjunctival surface uppermost onto a piece of card before fixation, this prevents it from curling up. Biopsy samples are usually taken from more than one site because the normal conjunctival morphology changes across the conjunctival sac.

Additional laboratory investigations

Serology may be useful in the investigation of some cases. Titers for feline herpesvirus and chlamydia may be an adjunct to the previously mentioned tests, depending on the vaccination status of the cat.

Table 7·2 Cellular response associated with specific conjunctivitis and keratitis [12].

Disease	Cellular response
Acute bacterial or fungal conjunctivitis	Predominantly neutrophils, few mononuclear cells; many bacteria or yeast/fungal elements; degenerating epithelial cells; RBCs may be present
Chronic bacterial or fungal conjunctivitis	Predominantly neutrophils, many mononuclear cells, degenerate or keratinized epithelial cells, goblet cells; bacteria may or may not be seen; mucus, fibrin present. Fungal or yeast elements are usually prominent in cell layers
Feline mycoplasma conjunctivitis	Predominantly neutrophils, fewer mononuclear cells, basophils; coccoid or pleomorphic organisms on cell membrane
Feline herpes viral conjunctivitis	Pseudomembrane formation, giant cells, multinucleated cells, fibrin, erythrocytes, neutrophils, and mononuclear cells (numbers depend on stage of infection); cell necrosis
Feline chlamydial conjunctivitis	Predominantly neutrophils; mononuclear cells in subacute cases are increased in number; plasma cells, basophilic cytoplasmic inclusions early in the disease
Keratoconjunctivitis sicca	Epithelial cells keratinized; goblet cells, mucus; neutrophilic response marked if there is much infection; bacteria present
Canine distemper	Varies with stage of disease (early: giant cells; later: neutrophils, goblet cells, and mucus). Infrequent intracellular inclusions; cell necrosis
Allergic conjunctivitis	Eosinophils; neutrophils may be marked; basophils possible
Bacterial/fungal keratitis	Predominantly neutrophils, degenerative epithelial cells. Bacterial organisms on surface of epithelial cells, neutrophils or intraepithelial; usually numerous fungal/yeast organisms

Treatment of conjunctivitis

Most conjunctival conditions can be treated adequately by topical drug administration; in some cases however systemic therapy may be useful. Subconjunctival injections are usually reserved for serious bacterial ulcers or intraocular infection.

Mild bacterial conjunctivitis in dogs is usually self-limiting and is generally treated by application of a broad-spectrum topical antibacterial preparation. Cases with severe or chronic conjunctivitis are worth investigating by taking swabs for bacteriology and scrapes for cytology. Initial antibacterial therapy can be chosen based on the Gram staining of smears while awaiting culture and sensitivity results. Mixed infections should initially be treated with a preparation with a broad-spectrum of activity such as a gramicidin, neomycin, and polymyxin B combination. Gentamicin, tobramycin, and cipro-floxacin have a broad spectrum of action against Gram- positive and -negative organisms, but are of particular use in the treatment of pseudomonal infections (often associated with progressive corneal ulcers). Where staphylococci are involved a drug such as fusidic acid can be effective. Long-term application of antibiotics in the absence of evidence of actual infection may lead to antibiotic resis-tance or overgrowth of organisms outside the spectrum of activity of the drug.

In cats, chlamydial infections respond to tetracyclines topically and systemically. Doxycycline is secreted in the tear film and is therefore a very good systemic adjunct to topical tetracyclines in these cases. In cases of FHV-1 infection topically applied antiviral preparations are used. It has been suggested from *in vitro* studies that trifluridine is the most effective topical agent, followed by idoxuridine, vidarabine, bromovinyldeoxyuridine, and lastly acyclovir [15]. However, in a recent clinical study a specific antiviral treatment that was clinically superior to other treatments could not be identified and results were poor [16].

Topical corticosteroids or cyclosporine are useful for treating immune-mediated conditions. Artificial tear solutions can be very effective in protecting the cornea where swelling prevents complete blinking and causes an exposure keratitis.

Dacryocystitis causing inflammatory discharge

Dacryocystitis is characterized by a profuse mucoid to mucopurulent ocular discharge which may be malodorous. The condition usually occurs unilaterally and involves the nasolacrimal excretory system and contiguous tissue [17]. Most cases are associated with foreign plant material. Treatment is aimed at removing any foreign material and irrigating the system. Usually the upper punctum is cannulated and sterile saline gently irrigated through it, some of the purulent material flushed out can be collected for culture and sensitivity. Care must be taken not to force any foreign bodies into the less acces-sible portions of the nasolacrimal duct. Enlarging the punctal open-ing by cutting open the conjunctival wall of the canaliculus (one blade of a pair of iris scissors is inserted into the punctum and the canaliculus wall is cut) may facilitate removal of foreign material in the lacrimal sac. Repeated flushing of the nasolacrimal system with an appropriate antibiotic solution may help control the infection and in non-responsive cases nasolacrimal catheterization is useful and has the added advantage of maintaining patency of the system. Catheterization is performed by passing monofilament nylon (0 or 2/0), the end of which has been blunted in a flame, from the upper punctum to the nasal ostium. Some manipulation may be required to encourage the monofilament nylon to exit from the nasal ostium. Polyethylene tubing (PE 50 or PE 90) of the required length is threaded over the monofilament nylon and hemostats used to grasp the nylon at either end. Gentle traction is applied to the distal hemostat and the tubing pulled through the system. Once the nasolacrimal system is catheterized the monofilament nylon is withdrawn and the ends of the catheter sutured at either end to the skin adjacent to the medial canthus and naris. The catheter is removed after about 3 weeks.

Sinus and orbital disease causing inflammatory discharge

Retrobulbar abscessation and orbital cellulitis will often cause marked conjunctival hyperemia, chemosis, and mucopurulent discharge. Zygomatic salivary gland mucocele occasionally results in swelling and discharge due to exposure of the conjunctiva. Ultrasound is very useful in the diagnosis and localization of orbital swellings and is used for guided biopsies of affected tissue (see p. 53–56). Extension of infection and neoplasia from the sinuses may give a similar presentation to retrobulbar abscessation. Retention mucocoeles in the frontal sinus can cause erosion of the frontal bone leading to recurrent drainage of accumulated secretions via the conjunctival sac. In addition to ultrasound, radiography, computerized tomography, and magnetic resonance imaging may provide useful diagnostic information. In all these cases culture and sensitivity is encouraged as are cytology and biopsy. Treatment is dependent on the etiology.

Other problems causing inflammatory discharge

Keratitis, either ulcerative, proliferative, or infectious is a common cause of ocular discharge. Problems which cause blepharitis may have conjunctival involvement. Immune-mediated diseases in dogs such as the pemphigus group and the uveodermatological syndrome can result in mucoid to mucopurulent ocular discharge. An ocular discharge may also accompany intraocular disease.

EPIPHORA (WATERY EYE) – AN OVERFLOW OF TEARS

Normal Drainage of Tears

Tears are constantly produced and are spread over the ocular surface by the action of the eyelids and third eyelid. Some evaporation of tears occurs, but the majority are removed from the ocular surface by drainage to the nasal chambers via the nasolacrimal duct (Figure 7.9). The proximal openings into the nasolacrimal drainage system consist of upper and lower puncta positioned just inside the lids, close to the medial canthus (Figure 7.10). These open into canaliculi which join forming the nasolacrimal duct. A slight dilation of the initial part of the duct is known as the lacrimal sac and is positioned in the lacrimal fossa at the nasoventral aspect of the orbital rim. Distal to the lacrimal sac the nasolacrimal duct passes through the lacrimal bone to run in a canal or groove on the medial surface of the maxilla. The duct opens on the lateral nasal floor and can be examined in dogs with a reasonable size of naris with the aid of a speculum. Some dogs, in particular brachycephalics, have an opening part way along the nasolacrimal duct in the posterior nasal cavity.

Tears enter the drainage system from the medial canthal lacrimal lake through the puncta into the canaliculi by capillary action. During

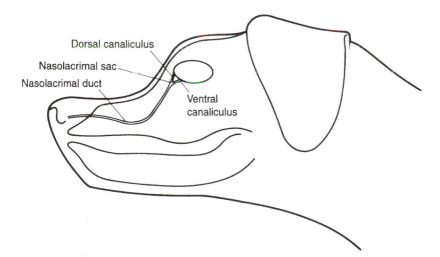

Figure 7.9 Diagram of the nasolacrimal system. (Redrawn with permission from the Post Graduate Foundation and Ms Rosemary Craig from Blogg JR and Stanley RG. Discharging Eye. In: *Common Eye Disease*, Proceedings 158, Post Graduate Committee in Veterinary Science, University of Sydney 1990: 223–236.)

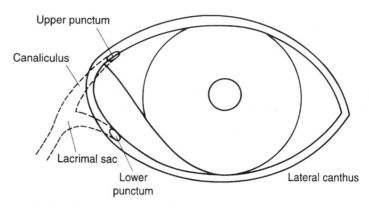

Figure 7.10   Diagram of the orbital portion of the nasolacrimal system. (Redrawn with permission from the Post Graduate Foundation and Ms Rosemary Craig from Blogg JR and Stanley RG. Discharging Eye. In: *Common Eye Disease*, Proceedings 158, Post Graduate Committee in Veterinary Science, University of Sydney 1990: 223–236.)

blinking closure of the puncta and compression of the canaliculi help to propel tears into the nasolacrimal duct. This is further aided by dilatation of the lacrimal sac creating a negative pressure and drawing tears into the sac. It is believed that there is a valve mechanism that stops the tears from refluxing from the nasolacrimal system back to the eye.

Examination of an animal with epiphora

Excessive tearing, or epiphora (tear overflow) [18], may reflect increased tear production as a result of ocular or nasal irritation or pain, or alternatively it may result from inadequate tear drainage, or possibly a combination of increased production and impaired drainage. Careful examination of the animal with epiphora should enable the veterinarian to decide if there is increased lacrimation due to irritation or pain. Initially the animal should be observed from a distance before stressing it by handling or placing on the examination table. This is important because an increased blink rate due to mild ocular irritation may not be exhibited once the animal is more closely restrained. Causes of ocular pain which may result in epiphora are considered in Chapter 6. Conditions more typically associated with irritation and epiphora are considered here as are problems relating to tear drainage.

Functional assessment of the nasolacrimal drainage system

Examination of the nasolacrimal drainage system aims to assess the overall process of tear drainage which consists of the physiological process of getting tears into the system as well as the actual anatomic patency of the system.

Direct examination

The external portion of the nasolacrimal drainage apparatus (the puncta) can be inspected by retracting the lid margins at the medial canthus. Magnification and good illumination facilitate the examination.

Fluorescein passage test

The passage of fluorescein dye from the ocular surface to the naris tests not only the patency of the system but also the overall process of tear drainage. In most normal dolichocephalic and mesocephalic breeds of dog fluorescein dye placed on the surface of the eye will reach the nares within 4 min. Use of a Wood's light highlights fluorescein at the nostril. The tongue should also be examined for fluorescein that may have exited by accessory openings of the nasolacrimal duct and drained via the nasopharynx. The fluorescein passage test may be negative in brachycephalics with patent nasolacrimal systems and in up to 50% of normal cats.

Nasolacrimal cannulation and irrigation

This investigation (Figure 7.11) is used to demonstrate anatomic patency of the system and is indicated should the fluorescein passage test be negative. Following topical anesthesia, and in most cats and some dogs sedation or even general anesthesia, the upper punctum is cannulated with a 20 to 24 gauge (27 gauge for cats) metal or plastic cannula (plastic nasolacrimal cannulae are easier to introduce if they are trimmed to about 5 mm in length with the tip cut obliquely) attached to a 5 ml syringe filled with sterile saline. As the system is flushed a stream of saline should exit through the lower punctum, if it is patent. To flush the remainder of the system the lower punctum is occluded by finger pressure. The flushing solution should then exit from the nose. Excessive flushing pressure should be avoided, particularly in cats and small breeds of dogs as it is possible to damage or even rupture the nasolacrimal system. If the presence of a foreign body is suspected take care not to force flush it further down the system.

When pus is flushed from the system either via the nose or punctum this indicates the presence of dacryocystitis (see above). If saline exits from the nose but the fluorescein passage test was slow or negative this may suggest that tears are not entering the system at a normal rate or drainage along it is impeded.

Cannulation of the nasolacrimal duct from the distal opening can

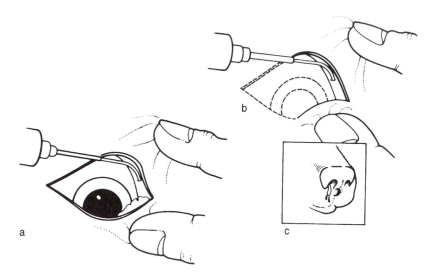

Figure 7.11   Flushing the nasolacrimal system. (a) Cannulate one of the puncta, gently irrigate and observe the flow of fluid through the other punctum, (b) occlude the other punctum and (c) watch for fluid passage through to the nose. Redrawn with permission from the Post Graduate Foundation and Ms Rosemary Craig from Blogg JR and Stanley RG. Discharging Eye. In: *Common Eye Disease*, Proceedings 158, Post Graduate Committee in Veterinary Science, University of Sydney 1990: 223–236.

be difficult, even in animals with reasonable sized nares. It may be attempted by dilation of the nostril with a speculum (an otoscope cone or a small dog sized vaginal speculum) or a pair of curved mosquito artery forceps. A monofilament suture is passed through the opening of the nasolacrimal duct (nasal ostium) on the lateral floor of the nasal cavity until it emerges from the upper punctum.

Radiography

Radiographic contrast solutions can be used to highlight the nasolacrimal system (dacryocystorhinography) and may help localize any blockage. Radiography can also be used to investigate causes of epiphora such as tooth root abscesses or neoplasia.

Epiphora associated with increased tear production

Increased tear production is due to reflex tearing in response to irritation of the ocular surface. The following conditions may cause epiphora:

Eyelid conditions:
- entropion (see p. 171–173)
- distichiasis ectopic cilia (see p. 174)
- trichiasis
- blepharitis (see p. 62–63)
- lid laceration
- neoplasia (see p. 62–63)

Third eyelid conditions:
- lymphoid hyperplasia
- prolapsed nictitans gland (may also interfere with drainage) (see p. 64)
- scrolled third eyelid (may also interfere with drainage) (see p. 63)

Ocular surface conditions:
- conjunctivitis (see above)
- keratitis (including ulceration)

Painful intraocular conditions (see Chapter 6)

Distichiasis

Distichiasis is very common in dogs. Distichia originate from follicles in or between the meibomian glands and exit from the eyelid along the eyelid margin, either through or adjacent to the meibomian ducts. Many dogs have distichiasis without showing clinical signs such as epiphora. This is because either the distichia do not contact the ocular surface, or they are fine and float in the precorneal tear film. In some cases where the distichia are large and stiff, a single distichium can irritate the eye producing epiphora and even corneal ulceration. Treatment consists of destruction or removal of the offending follicles. Destruction is achieved by electrolysis or cryoepilation. Various lid splitting techniques have been described but should only be used with the aid of magnification as if they are inexpertly performed they can result in problems due to eyelid scarring and distortion.

Trichiasis

Trichiasis is a condition in which normally positioned hairs contact the cornea. Facial hair may act as an irritant in breeds such as the Pekinese, Poodle, and Lhasa Apso. Trichiasis from the nasal fold, the medial canthus, or the caruncle is a common cause of epiphora in breeds of dog such as Pekinese, Bulldog, and the Pug. Affected dogs often develop a medial pigmentary keratitis. Application of petroleum jelly to the hair of the nasal fold gives temporary relief and can be used for those dogs intended for the show ring. In severely affected dogs the nasal fold or the hairy caruncle can be surgically excised or a generous medial canthorrhaphy performed to protect the cornea. Removal of nasal folds is quite straightforward, once the surgical site is clipped the fold requiring removal is obvious. Hair at the medial canthus or the caruncle is removed by dissecting the hair-bearing tissue from the conjunctiva and lid margin with fine scissors (magnification is required) taking care not to injure the puncta. Cryosurgical treatment has also been described as a treatment for this problem.

Upper eyelid entropion/trichiasis is considered on pp. 173–174.

Epiphora associated with impaired tear drainage

Congenital or conformational causes of impaired tear drainage

Decreased tear drainage may be due to a congenital absence of the punctum, canaliculi, and/or nasolacrimal ducts and will cause epiphora. Atresia of the lower punctum is the most common congenital cause in dogs, in particular the Golden Retriever and English Cocker Spaniel. This condition is readily corrected as follows: first insert a 20 to 22 guage cannula into the patent punctum (in most cases the upper one), then flush to elevate the conjunctiva over the canaliculus adjacent to the occluded punctum. An opening is made into the canaliculus by excising a small piece of overlying conjunctiva. Some cats present with imperforate puncta; in contrast to dogs the upper punctum is more commonly affected than the lower.

A less common cause of epiphora is the congenital displacement of the punctum from its normal palpebral site to another position on the eyelid. The punctum may also be displaced by entropion or ectropion.

Epiphora resulting in a red-brown staining of facial hair below the medial canthus is common in breeds such as Miniature Poodles, Toy Poodles, Shih Tzu, and Maltese. It is most apparent in dogs with a light colored coat and is primarily a cosmetic problem. However, dermatitis may develop under the stained hair. In affected breeds a prominent globe, shallow medial canthal lake, and tight lower lid to globe apposition result in suboptimal tear drainage [23]. Accompanying conditions include medial entropion which functionally occludes the punctum and long medial canthal hairs which lie in the tear film and act as a 'wick' along which tears pass onto the face. It is possible that the staining of the facial hairs is due to porphyrins in the tears. In many cases the tear staining is difficult to eliminate completely. Any obvious causes of the epiphora need to be treated, e.g. blocked nasolacrimal ducts. Flushing of the nasolacrimal ducts, correction of medial entropion, and removal of hair-bearing medial canthal tissue may assist in the management of the condition. Medial entropion of the lower eyelid may be corrected by an adaptation of the standard entropion correction in which a triangular-shaped piece of skin is excised adjacent to the offending portion of eyelid and the defect repaired with fine sutures taking care that the knots do not irritate the eye [24]. Many Persian cats also suffer from epiphora and tear staining, and this is probably related to extreme deformity of the nasolacrimal system coupled to the prominent globes and shallow medial canthal lakes. Often little can be done to resolve this largely cosmetic problem. The use of potentially caustic cleaning agents such as peroxides to treat tear staining should be discouraged.

Acquired causes of impaired tear drainage

An acquired blockage of the puncta and canaliculi is seen in young cats following symblepharon formation as a result of feline herpesvirus infection. The puncta may be occluded by overlying scarred conjunctiva, or the canaliculi themselves may be scarred by the viral infection. Surgery to remove the conjunctival adhesions does not seem to be effective in reducing the epiphora.

Scarring as a result of injury and the presence of medially positioned eyelid tumors may potentially impair tear drainage. Neoplasms involving the nasal cavity, sinuses, or medial canthal area may also cause epiphora. Neoplasia of the nasolacrimal ducts is rare. Obstructions of the nasolacrimal duct most commonly result from infection, usually associated with a foreign body. Removal of nasolacrimal foreign bodies and nasolacrimal catheterization are discussed on p. 209–210.

When patency of the drainage system cannot be reestablished the epiphora may be resolved by creating an artificial nasolacrimal duct. Epiphora is generally a cosmetic problem so it is debatable whether this surgery is justifiable. Also the procedures to create a new duct are involved and should only be considered as a final option. Two techniques have been described [25, 26]. Referral to a veterinary eye specialist is recommended.

Lacerations involving the nasolacrimal system

Any injury in the area of the medial canthus may potentially involve the nasolacrimal system. The puncta and canaliculi need to be identified and cannulated prior to suturing. The cannulae should be left in place during the healing period [27].

REDUCED OR ALTERED TEAR PRODUCTION

This section considers keratoconjunctivitis sicca (KCS) which is a condition resulting from a deficiency of aqueous tears that occurs commonly in dogs and infrequently in cats. Other forms of ocular surface disease resulting from an altered tear film also occur, but these are far less common and even less often recognized. They are considered at the end of this chapter.

Reduced aqueous tear production (keratoconjunctivitis sicca)

Clinical signs

KCS in the dog is most commonly a chronic progressive disorder. It may be unilateral or bilateral. Dogs with a moderately lowered tear production may present with a chronic or recurrent conjunctivitis and minimal corneal involvement. The diagnosis is not always obvious at this stage and a Schirmer tear test should be performed on all dogs with this presentation. As the tear production further decreases and the condition progresses it is typified in the dog by an accumulation of tacky mucoid or mucopurulent discharge (Figure 7.12). The discharge clings to the conjunctival fornices and corneal surface and may stick the eyelids together. The conjunctiva becomes hyperemic, thickened, and possibly pigmented. There is a lack of corneal lustre accompanied by a variable degree of superficial vascularization, pigmentation, and scarring (Figure 7.13). Some animals also have a dry nostril on the affected side. There is a variable amount of resultant discomfort or pain but some degree of blepharospasm is

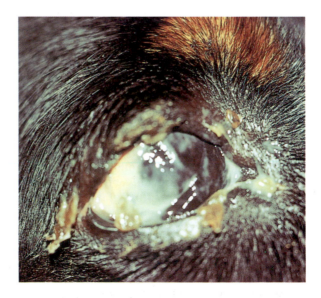

Figure 7.12   Tacky mucopurulent discharge in a dog with KCS.

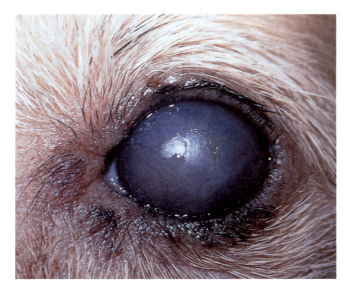

Figure 7.13 Dull cornea with signs of KCS.

usual. Corneal ulceration develops in some cases, particularly those with an acute onset. The ulceration may be progressive, possibly leading to descemetocele formation or perforation. Secondary bacterial involvement exacerbates the problem.

There is a marked breed incidence for KCS and predisposed breeds include West Highland White terrier, Cocker spaniel, Shihtzu, Lhasa Apso, Cavalier King Charles spaniel, Bull Terrier, Bulldog, Miniature Schnauzer, Dachshund, Chihuahua, and Pekinese. The frequency of KCS within each breed appears to vary from country to country. A positive interaction between age and gender on occurrence of KCS exists [28]. Older dogs are more predisposed than younger ones and neutered animals are more predisposed than intact males and females. The incidence of KCS is higher in dogs with low androgen levels.

Keratoconjunctivitis sicca also occurs in the cat albeit far less commonly. In contrast to the dog, the resultant ocular discharge is minimal and corneal changes develop much more slowly.

Pathogenesis of KCS

- *KCS apparent at the time of eyelid opening.* This may be due to congenital hypoplasia of the lacrimal gland or a retarded functional development of the tear producing glands. Tear production can increase to normal levels in the latter case.
- *Autoimmune adenitis of glandular tissue* [29]. The majority of

cases of canine KCS probably fall into this category. Histology of the lacrimal gland reveals breakup of glandular structure with duct dilation and epithelial cell loss, mononuclear cell infiltration, and fibrosis.

- *Trauma.* KCS due to trauma may be the result of damage to the parasympathetic supply to the lacrimal glands. In some instances normal lacrimal secretion may return over 1–2 months.
- *Neurogenic KCS* results from denervation of the tear producing glands. Causes include trauma, infection, neoplasia, and surgical intervention. The ipsilateral nostril may also be dry. Lesions which also involve the motor branch of the facial nerve (VII) result in facial paralysis, including an inability to blink.
- *Iatrogenic* causes include gland intoxication by some sulfa drugs, e.g. sulfadiazine, sulfasalazine [30] and trimethoprim/sulfamethoxazole [31]. Atropine and atropine-like substances reduce tear production [32] and local and general anesthesia results in decreased tear volume [33]. Acute KCS may therefore follow a surgical procedure where atropine and general anesthesia have been given. Surgical removal of accessory lacrimal gland tissue in the third eyelid, e.g. cherry eye excision, can lead to KCS later in life [34].
- *KCS secondary to chronic conjunctivitis* with obstruction of secretory ductules. A common example of this is the older Cocker spaniel with upper lid entropion/trichiasis and chronic keratoconjunctivitis. Correction of the eyelid disorder, with treatment for KCS, usually leads to a return of normal lacrimal function. KCS in the cat sometimes follows feline herpes virus infection
- *Distemper-associated KCS* [35]. Distemper can cause a dacryoadenitis with resultant destruction of the glandular tissue.

Diagnosis

The diagnosis is based upon clinical signs and the result of the Schirmer tear test (STT) (Figure 7.3). The normal tear production of the dog results in a STT reading in excess of 15 mm min^{-1} wetting [36] while that of the normal cat exceeds 10 mm min^{-1} [37]. Readings of less than 10 mm min^{-1} in the dog and less than 5 mm min^{-1} in the cat indicate a lack of tear production and probable KCS.

Management of KCS

Medical therapy

The majority of cases of KCS can be managed medically and parotid duct transposition is now less frequently performed than in the past. The initial STT reading has some prognostic value; generally speaking the lower the level and the more long-standing the condition, the less likely it is that treatment will result in a great increase in tear production, although in some instances dogs initially presenting with STT readings of $0\,\mathrm{mm}\ \mathrm{min}^{-1}$ do show dramatic increases in tear production.

Stimulation of tear production can be achieved, in many cases, by the use of twice daily topical cyclosporine ophthalmic ointment (Optimmune, Schering-Plough Animal Health Corp.) [38]. Where the commercial preparation is not available a 1–2% solution of cyclosporine (Sandimmune for oral administration, Sandoz Pharmaceuticals) in a vegetable oil, such as corn oil has been used. Cyclosporine not only stimulates tear production and modulates any inflammatory reaction within the lacrimal tissue but it also slowly reverses some of the corneal changes. Prior to the introduction of cyclosporine, topical corticosteroid preparations were often used with similar intention, although obviously not in ulcerated eyes. In-between administration of cyclosporine, an artificial tear preparation should be instilled into the eye at a frequency commensurate with the degree of dryness. The owners should also be shown how gently to clean the eye of any accumulated discharges. Additional therapy includes application of a lubricating ointment last thing at night. This author favors a corticosteroid-containing ointment which will also serve to reduce inflammation, but should be avoided if there is corneal ulceration. The use of oral pilocarpine, 1–4 drops of a 1% ophthalmic solution disguised in food, can stimulate tear production, especially in animals with neurogenic KCS and resulting denervation hypersensitivity.

The medical regimes described above can be time consuming and may not be possible for some owners. In these cases expect poor therapeutic results.

Repeat STTs are performed monthly to assess any improvement in wetting. It may take up to 6 weeks to see an improvement in STT reading. However, even when STT levels remain low there is usually some alleviation of discomfort and improvement in clinical signs with this treatment regime. Most dogs with KCS are likely to require long-term treatment and this fact should be emphasized to the owners.

Surgical procedures employed in the management of KCS

Brachycephalics in particular may benefit from a lateral tarsorraphy to shorten the palpebral fissure and thus reduce the evaporative surface of the cornea [38]. Dogs which develop corneal ulceration require specific therapy including topical antibiotics, and for deep or deepening ulcers application of conjunctival flaps to prevent perforation.

Transposition of the parotid salivary duct papilla to the conjunctival fornix provides salivary lubrication for the eye and is restricted to those

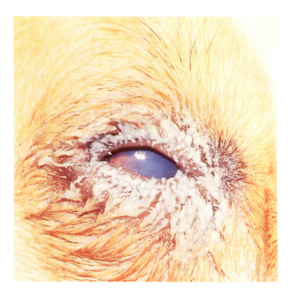

Figure 7.14   Salivary salts precipitated around eyelids of a dog after parotid duct transposition.

cases where the disease cannot be controlled medically [39]. Parotid saliva is physiologically similar to tears in pH, osmolarity, and immunoglobulin concentrations and can act satisfactorily as a tear substitute. Parotid duct transposition (PDT) is less commonly required now due to the recent advances in medical therapy. Generally speaking in animals suffering from neurogenic KCS parotid salivary secretion is unaffected because the parotid innervation is via the glossopharyngeal nerve (IXth cranial nerve) whereas the lacrimal gland innervation is via the facial nerve (VIIth cranial nerve). PDT is not without potential complications. These include over wetting of the eye and face with saliva and the precipitation of salivary salts on lid margins and the corneal surface (Figure 7.14). The salivary overflow can result in blepharitis and the precipitates tend to irritate the eye. Emollients and chelation with EDTA solutions seldom ease the irritation. Postoperative complications, if severe, may necessitate reversal of the procedure. PDT is possible but rarely required in the cat.

Ocular surface disease resulting from inadequate distribution of the tear film

Inadequate blinking or eyelid closure can result in a breakup of the tear film over the central cornea with dry spot formation and the development of an exposure keratopathy. This may result from the anatomic characteristics of the animal, from exophthalmos, as a result

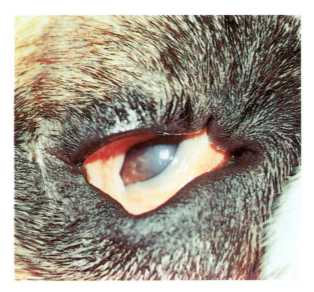

Figure 7.15   Eyelid deformity in a giant breed of dog.

of congenital or acquired eyelid deformity, or as a result of reduced blinking due to sensory or motor deficits:

- A wide palpebral fissure and loose lower lid reduce effective eyelid closure, so that the spreading of a tear film and cleaning of the cornea are impaired (Figure 7.15).
- Brachycephalic breeds often have a long palpebral fissure, prominent globe, and limited third eyelid movement which predisposes them to corneal pathology resulting from inadequacy of tear film function.
- Exophthalmos due to orbital space-occupying lesions can result in an inability to close the eyelids leading to corneal pathology.
- Colobomatous congenital eyelid defects and acquired eyelid defects can also prevent adequate corneal coverage by the lids. Cicatricial contraction of eyelid wounds can lead to keratitis in a defined area. Iatrogenic eyelid dysfunction is commonest as a result of overzealous entropion repair. Surgical correction of such deformity is usually successful.
- A lack of blink due to impaired facial nerve (CN VII) function may be of central or peripheral origin. The location of the lesion is critical to prognosis and treatment [40]. The maintenance of a healthy cornea relies upon the effectiveness of the third eyelid in cleaning the cornea and spreading a tear film. Where the nictitans has limited movement (brachycephalics, exophthalmos, reduced

retractor oculi muscle function, or innervation), discharge, corneal clouding and possibly ulceration will result.

- Inadequate corneal sensation due to lesions involving the ophthalmic division of the trigeminal (V) nerve typically results in ulceration of the portion of cornea exposed within the palpebral fissure. This is partly due to reduced blinking and therefore inadequate spreading of the tear film.

Qualitative tear film disease

As well as disease resulting from inadequate production of aqueous tears or inadequate distribution of the produced tears, changes in either the lipid or mucus phases of the tear film can also cause ocular surface disease. These conditions are rarely diagnosed.

A deficiency of goblet cells leads to instability of the tear film [41]. This results in a superficial keratitis in the presence of adequate aqueous tears. There is also a notable lack of mucus associated with the ocular discharge. An assessment of the tear breakup (BUT) time will determine adequacy of tear film mucins [2, 42]. A fluorescein stain BUT is assessed by holding the lids open after applying fluorescein to the tear film and observing the eye under a cobalt blue light looking for the first sign of tear breakup which is seen as the formation of a dark spot. Normal BUT is approximately 20 s. Mucin-deficiency BUT is < 5 s [41, 42]. Conjunctival biopsy will record markedly reduced goblet cell numbers.

Chronic eyelid disease and meibomian gland inflammation may reduce production of the lipid phase of the tear film resulting in tear film instability and ocular surface disease. Lipid layer assessment requires specialist equipment which is not widely available but suspicion increases with lid margin disease or meibomian adenitis where acini are blocked with white oily secretion.

REFERENCES

1. Lemp MA and Wolfley DE. The lacrimal apparatus. In: Hart WM (ed) *Adler's Physiology of the Eye*, 9th edn. St Louis: Mosby-Year Book 1992: 18–28.
2. Moore CP, Wilsman NJ, Nordheim EV, Majors LJ and Collier LL Density and distribution of canine conjunctival goblet cells. *Invest. Ophthalmol. Vis. Sci.* 1987; **28**: 1925–32.
3. Gaskin JM. Microbiology of the canine and feline eye. *Vet. Clin. North. Am. (Small Anim. Pract.)* 1980; **10**: 303–16.
4. Samuelson DA, Andresen TL and Gwin RM. Conjunctival fungal flora in horses, cattle, dogs and cats. *J. Am. Vet. Med. Assoc.* 1984; **184**: 1240–2.
5. Peng CG and Jiang JS. Treatment of ocular thelaziasis in dogs. *Chin. J. Vet. Med.* 1983; **9**:18–9.

6. Glaze MB. Ocular allergy. *Semin. Vet. Med. and Surg. (Small Anim.)*, 1991; **6**: 296–302.
7. Brooks DE. Canine conjunctiva and nictitating membrane. In: Gelatt KN (ed) *Veterinary Ophthalmology* 2nd edn. Philadephia: Lea and Febiger 1990: 290–306.
8. Paulsen ME, Lavach JD, Snyder SP, Severn GA and Eichenbaum JD Nodular granulomatous episclerokeratitis in dogs: 19 cases (1973–1985). *J. Am. Vet. Med. Ass.* 1987; **190**: 1581–7.
9. Nasisse MP. Manifestations, diagnosis and treatment of ocular herpesvirus infection in the cat. *Comp. Cont. Educ. Pract. Vet.* 1982; **4**: 962–70.
10. Nasisse MP. Feline ophthalmology. In: Gelatt KN (ed) *Veterinary Ophthalmology* 2nd edn. Philadephia: Lea and Febiger 1990: 529–75.
11. Pentlarge VW. Eosinophilic conjunctivitis in five cats. *J. Am. Anim. Hosp. Ass.* 1991; **27**: 21–8.
12. Murphy JM. Exfoliative cytologic examination as an aid in diagnosing ocular diseases in the dog and cat. *Semin. in. Vet. Med. Surg. (Small Anim.)* 1988; 3: 10-4.
13. Valencia M. Contribution to the study of canine distemper. 1. Direct immunofluorscence and detection of inclusion bodies in live animal smears. *Medicina Veterinaria* 1987; **4**: 211–8.
14. Nasisse MP, Guy JS, Stevens JB, English RV and Davidson MG. Clinical and laboratory findings in chronic conjunctivitis in cats: 91 cases (1983–1991). *J. Am. Vet. Med. Ass.* 1993; **203**: 834–7.
15. Nasisse MP, Guy JS, Davidson MG, English RV and Davidson MG. In vitro susceptibility of feline herpesvirus-1 to vidarabine, idoxuridine, trifluridine, acyclovir, or bromovinyldeoxyuridine. *Am. J. Vet. Res.* 1989; **50**: 158–60.
16. Stiles J. Treatment of cats with ocular disease attributable to herpesvirus infection: 17 cases (1983–1993). *J. Am. Vet. Med. Ass.* 1995; **207**: 599–603.
17. Lavach JD, Severin GA and Roberts SM. Dacryocystitis in dogs: A review of twenty two cases. *J. Am. Anim. Hosp. Ass.* 1984; **20**: 463–7.
18. Habin D. The nasolacrimal system. In: Petersen-Jones SM & Crispin SM (eds) *Manual of Small Animal Ophthalmology*, Cheltenham: British Small Animal Veterinary Association 1993: 91–102.
19. Wheeler CA and Severin GA. Cryosurgical epilation for the treatment of distichiasis in the dog and cat. *J. Am. Anim. Hosp. Ass.* 1984; **20**: 877–84.
20. Halliwell WH. Surgical management of canine distichia. *J. Am. Vet. Med Ass.* 1967; **150**: 892–7.
21. Bedford PGC. Distichiasis and its treatment by method of partial tarsal plate excision. *J. Small Anim. Pract.* 1973; **14**: 1–7.
22. Barnett KC. Imperforate and micro-lachrymal puncta in the dog. *J. Small Anim. Pract.* 1978; **19**: 481–90.
23. Gelatt KN. Canine lacrimal and nasolacrimal systems. In: Gelatt KN (ed) *Veterinary Ophthalmology* 2nd edn. Philadelphia: Lea and Febiger, 1991: 276–89.
24. Peifffer Rl, Gelatt KN and Gwin RM. Correction of inferior medial entropion as a cause of epiphora. *Canine Pract.* 1978; **5**: 27–31.

25. Long R. Relief of epiphora by conjunctivorhinostomy. *J. Small Anim. Pract.* 1975; **16**: 381–6.
26. Covitz D, Hunziker J and Koch SA. Conjunctivohinostomy: A surgical method for the control of epiphora in the dog and cat. *J. Am. Vet. Med. Ass.* 1977; **171**: 251–5.
27. Lavach JD The lacrimal system. In: Slatter D (ed) *Textbook of Small Animal Surgery*, 2nd edn. Philadelphia: WB Saunders 1993 1184–94.
28. Kaswan RL, Salisbury MA and Lothrop CD. Interaction of age and gender on occurrence of canine keratoconjunctivitis sicca. *Prog. Vet. Comp. Ophthalmol.* 1991; **1**: 93–7.
29. Kaswan RL, Martin CL and Dawe DL. Keratoconjunctivitis sicca: Immunological evaluation of 62 canine cases. *Am. J. Vet. Res.* 1985; **46**: 376–83.
30. Slatter DH and Blogg JR. Keratoconjunctivitis sicca in dogs associated with sulphonamide administration. *Aust. Vet. J.* 1978; **54**: 444–6.
31. Morgan RV and Bachrach A. Keratoconjunctivitis sicca associated with sulphonamide therapy in dogs. *J. Am. Vet. Med. Ass.* 1982; **180**: 432–4.
32. Ludders JW and Heavner JE. Effect of atropine on tear formation in anaesthetized dogs. *J. Am. Vet. Med. Ass.* 1979; **175**: 585–6.
33. Vestre WA Brightman AH, Helper LC, and Lowery JC. Decreased tear production associated with general anaesthesia in the dog. *J. Am. Vet. Med. Ass.* 1979; **174**: 1006–7.
34. Morgan RV. To excise or not to excise. *Prog. Vet. Comp. Ophthalmol.* 1993; **3**: 109–10.
35. Martin CL and Kaswan R. Distemper-associated keratoconjunctivitis sicca. *J. Am. Anim. Hosp. Ass.* 1985; **21**: 355–9.
36. Rubin LF, Lynch RK and Stockman WS. Clinical estimation of lacrimal function in dogs. *J. Am. Vet. Med. Ass.* 1965; **147**: 946–7.
37. Veith LA, Cure TH and Gelatt KN. The Schirmer tear test in cats. *Mod. Vet. Pract.* 1970; **51**: 48–9.
38. Kaswan RL. A new perspective on canine keratoconjunctivitis sicca. *Vet. Clin. North Am. (Small Anim. Pract.)* 1990; **20**: 583–613.
39. Severin GA. Keratoconjunctivitis sicca. *Vet. Clin. North Am. (Small Anim. Pract.)* 1973; **3**: 407–22.
40. Scagliotti RH. Neuro-ophthalmology. In : Gelatt KN (ed) *Veterinary Ophthalmology* 2nd edn. Philadelphia: Lea and Febiger 1991: 706–43.
41. Moore CP and Collier LL. Ocular surface disease associated with loss of conjunctival goblet cells in dogs. *J. Am. Anim. Hosp. Assoc.* 1990; **26**: 458–66.
42. Moore CP. Qualitative tear film disease. *Vet. Clin. N. Am. (Small Anim. Pract.)* 1990; **20**: 565–81.

Index

Note – Page numbers in italic refer to illustrations and tables: **bold** page numbers indicate a main discussion